Healing Pretty

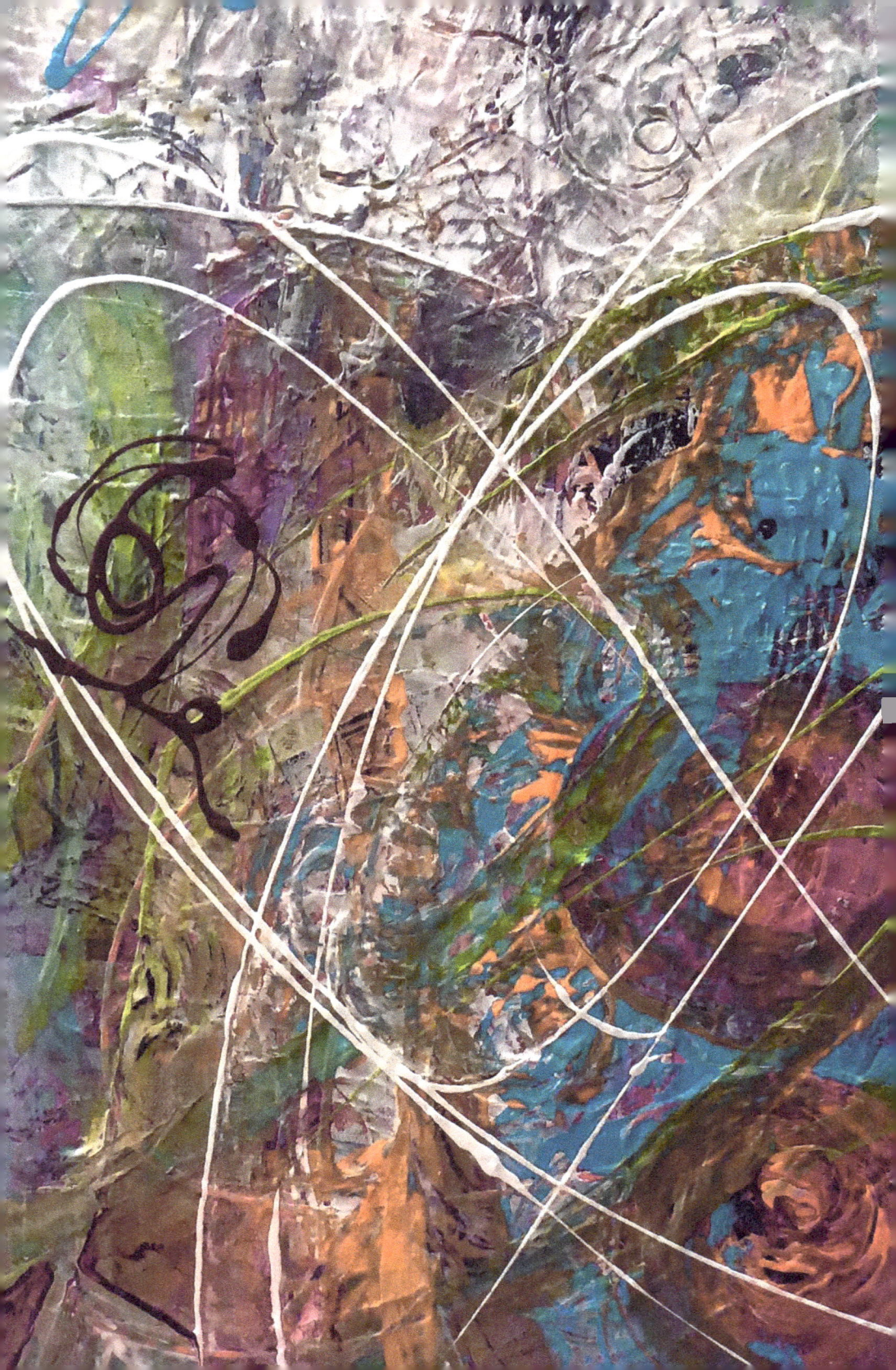

Praise for

Healing Pretty

"*Healing Pretty* is a heartwarming, inspiring, and uplifting read. It's easy to understand, with great tips to keep women feeling beautiful during their battle with cancer. The attention to sanitation and preventing infection made me confident that I can recommend this to my patients. Thank you, Jackie, for helping women find strength and camaraderie when they need it most." –*Jennifer Nadalin, BScN, RN, CONC*

"Engaging. Empowering. Enlightening. Three words that not only describe *Healing Pretty* but also the author. Her passion and commitment to those diagnosed with cancer are evident in all that she does. *Healing Pretty* is a warm, big, loving hug! It allows the reader to feel like someone is there for them and understands what they are going through. Thank you, Jackie, for loving patients through it!" –*Houida Kassem, Executive Director of Windsor Cancer Centre Foundation*

"*Healing Pretty* is a wonderful and informative resource for our patients. Thank you for this work, Jackie." –*Monica Staley Liang, RN, BScN, LLB, Regional Vice President Cancer Services, Windsor Regional Hospital*

"When my best friend was diagnosed, I reached out to Jackie who gave me a pre-release copy of *Healing Pretty*. I made a list of all the resources and put together a gift basket of the recommended skin-care lotions, candies, and comfort accessories. It made me feel great that I could do something meaningful for my best friend. *Healing Pretty* was a godsend." –*Kelly Vadnais*

"Where do I go from here, what information do I need, how do I go about finding it? *Healing Pretty* brought peace to my troubled mind, providing information and resources such as websites, wig options, prosthetics, and products to ease my way on this journey, plus the women who so graciously shared their stories, and so much more. Thank you, Jackie, for empowering all the women who will read this book." —*Tracey Stevenson, cancer warrior*

"Thank you for providing something that is lighthearted, complete, honest, and informative. *Healing Pretty* explores a variety of cancers that many women will relate to based on their own diagnosis." —*Daniella Czudner, cancer warrior*

"Your medical team gives you all the information they have, but it's the little things in between, like what do I do when my hair falls out? Do I just let it all fall out, or do I shave it? What am I going to do without breasts? It's all the little things we take for granted every single day that suddenly become such a huge part of your life. The focus was I need to get better, but how do I not lose myself in the process? When I was diagnosed at only 23 years old, I wish I'd had this book." —*Jill Laframboise, cancer warrior*

"The number one issue women and their caregivers shared was the lack of information on what to expect. They also lacked credible sources for tools and resources to cope with many of the esthetic and related side effects. *Healing Pretty* bridges the information gaps and provides trustworthy and reliable information, and all in one place. This invites women to be active participants in their own care, eases their anxiety, and contributes to better health outcomes." —*Cathy Mombourquette, former Cancer Care Ontario Regional Cancer Program Patient-Centred Care Lead, and Patient & Family Advisory Council Chair*

"*Healing Pretty* was honestly the best gift I received during my treatment. I'm not a reader, and I was terrified of what I found on the Internet, so this book kept it simple and to the point without all the medical terms and confusing lingo. It was light reading so I could read while waiting for appointments, and it gave me all the tools I needed to help me through my treatment process."
–Rachel Spadotto, cancer warrior

"*Healing Pretty* is FABULOUS! It will definitely be my go-to gift for women going through cancer treatment. It is so practical and well laid out. Congratulations to all involved!"
–Karen Metcalfe, Assistant Director, WE-SPARK Health Institute

"This is the best gift you can get someone with cancer. I gave a pre-release copy to my girlfriend who was just diagnosed. *Healing Pretty* helped her every day in her struggle to understand her life now, and helped her get back her self-esteem and self-worth."*–Catherine Murphy*

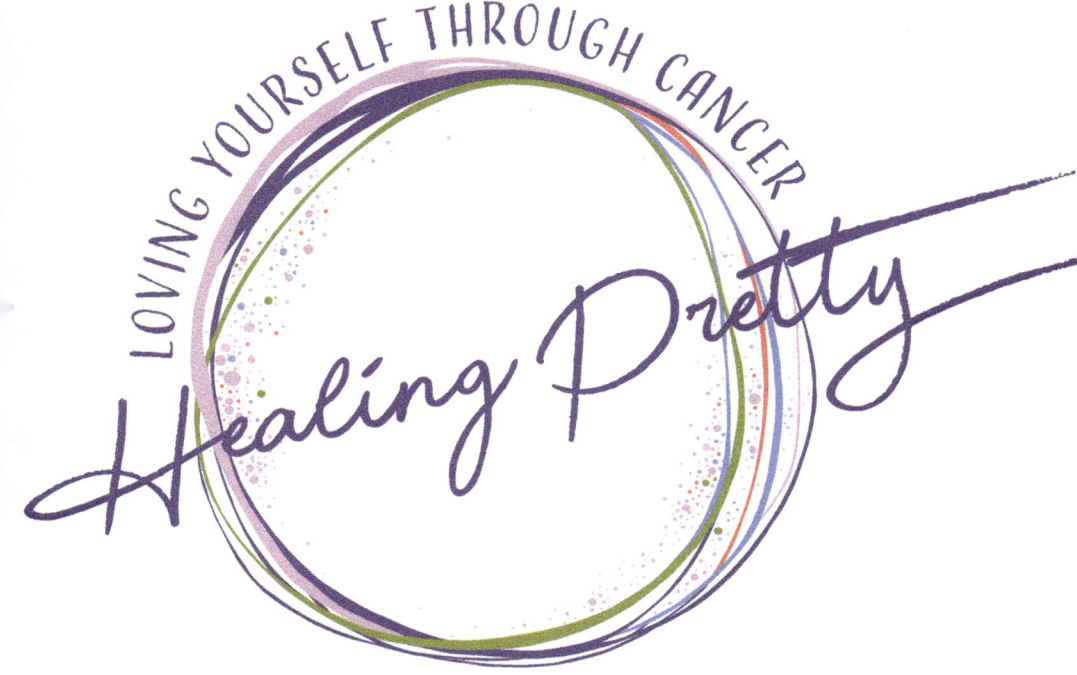

LOVING YOURSELF THROUGH CANCER

Healing Pretty

THE ULTIMATE GUIDE
TO FEELING COMFORTABLE,
CONFIDENT AND IN CONTROL
THROUGHOUT CANCER

JACQUELINE APOSTOL-PIZZUTI

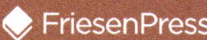 FriesenPress

Suite 300 - 990 Fort St
Victoria, BC, V8V 3K2 Canada
www.friesenpress.com

ISBN
978-1-5255-5448-3 (Hardcover)
978-1-5255-5449-0 (Paperback)
978-1-5255-5450-6 (eBook)

Health & Fitness, Diseases, Cancer

Artwork:
Marie Prevoo
mariesart@yahoo.ca
Facebook: MariesArt by Marie Prevoo

Healing Pretty Logo & Website:
Tianna Marie, LLC Creative Studio
www.tiannamarie.com

Photos of Author & Soul Sisters:
Mike LePine Photography
Instagram: @lepine_photography

Ordering Information:
Special discounts are available on
quantity purchases by individuals and
organizations. Please contact:
Jackie@healingprettybook.com
www.healingprettybook.com

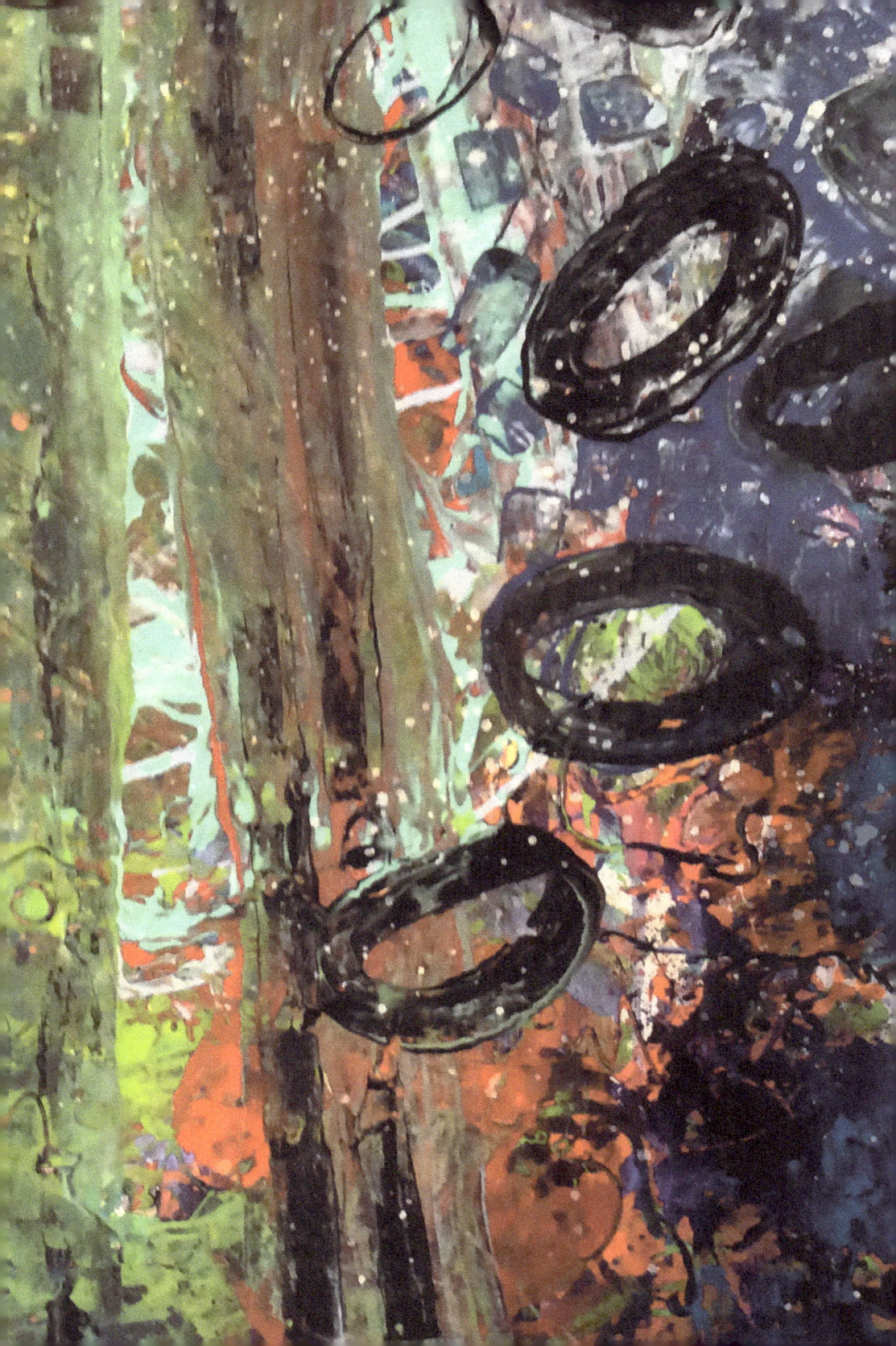

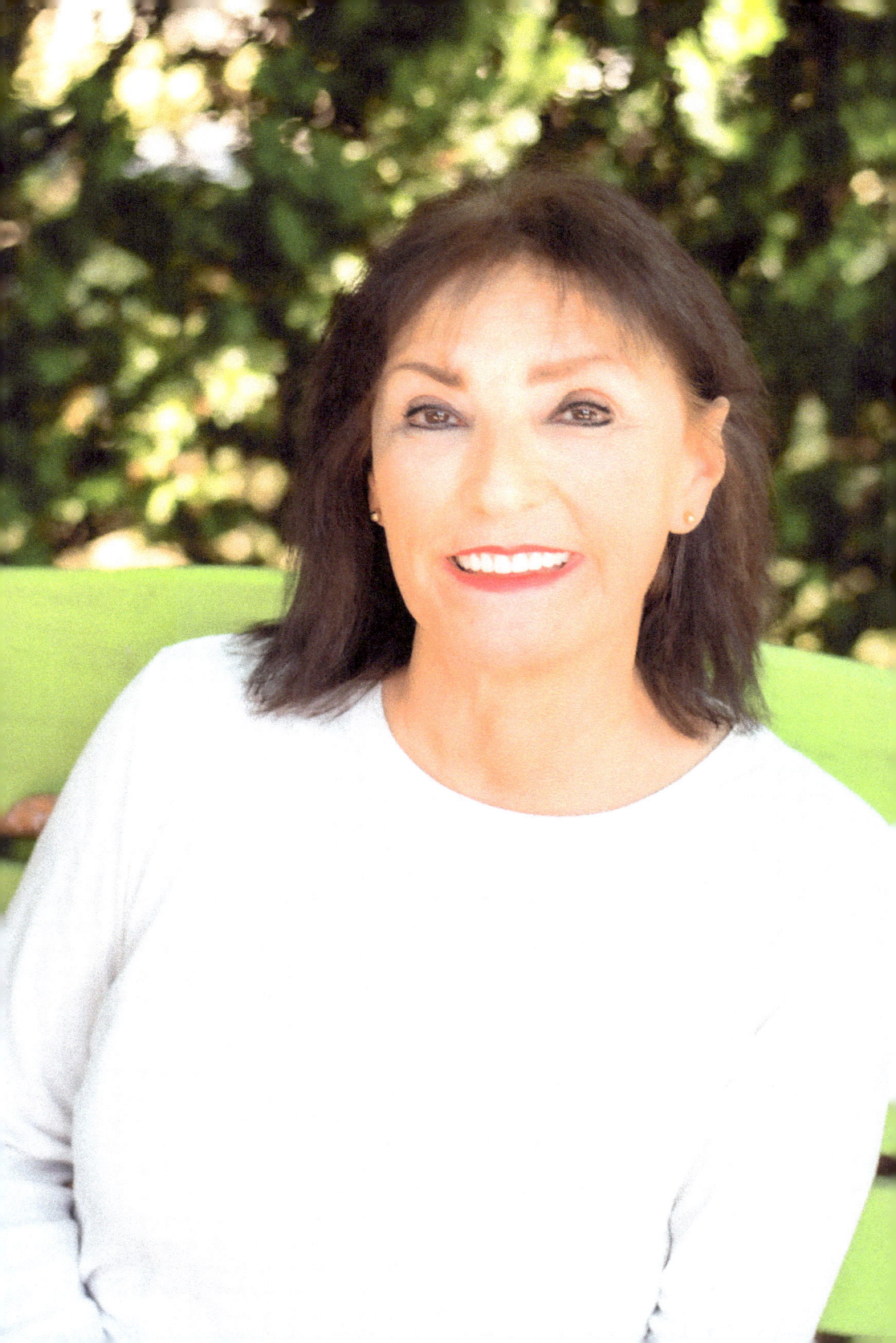

Dedication

In 1998, my sister Annette was diagnosed with lung cancer that had metastasized to her brain. She was given a fifteen percent chance of survival.

Twenty years later, my dear sister's cancer returned, and because of other complications, she passed away. However, although the cancer returned, in some sense, I believe it didn't win.

Annette was always there for me, as well as for our siblings, our parents, and so many friends. We could always count on her for support, encouragement, and kindness.

She has been with me since the inception of *Healing Pretty*. She was excited to be a part of it, and as always, she was eager to help in any way. This photo was taken only four months prior to her passing. She never let on that she wasn't feeling well.

I ask you to share with me in honoring my sister's memory. A remarkable woman of strength, courage, compassion, and grace, let her be your inspiration to fight and conquer with dignity.

In loving memory of my beloved big sister Annette, I dedicate this book to her.

Anastasia Clara Apostol

July 22, 1956–January 19, 2018

In the fall of 2018, I had a fundraising campaign to help provide free copies of *Healing Pretty* to those who were financially disadvantaged and to cancer care organizations.

I am so very grateful to all the people who supported my campaign. One of the reward levels was to have a personalized dedication appear in the book. Thank you to these wonderful people:

- Jack and Diane Apostol, "To our loving daughter Annette."
- Theresa Balaz, "To Dave Smith."
- Sheila Blair Mosley
- Linda Crowley, "To Leslie Byrne, who continues the fight."
- Claudia den Boer, "In memory of my dear friend Rosemary Limarzi."
- Eileen Ehrlich, "To Jackie, and all of the ladies who contributed or worked so hard on *Healing Pretty*."
- Erin Mammarella, "To all the healers, support people, and most of all, to Jackie for providing *Healing Pretty*. It takes a village to support cancer warriors!"
- Sheila Moroun
- Dana Mulholland, "To the Mulholland and Chevalier families."
- Rona Paquette, "To Jackie Apostol."
- Maria Peagler, "To Mary Lula Pickren."
- Janis Rosenberg
- Rachel Spadotto, "To my mom, Sheila Couvillon, who has been battling lung and skin cancer."
- Pamela Taylor, "In honor of my sweet Jill Laframboise."
- Jackie Roy, "To my aunts Lorraine Ruta and Rita Terry, and to Rita's daughter Jo-Anne."

This book is also dedicated to the loving memory of the generous and courageous Soul Sisters, Sonia Coletti and Kathy McIntyre, who have passed since the first edition of *Healing Pretty*.

"You can do it. You can get through this. One step at a time."

—Amy Robach, television presenter for ABC News, co-anchor of 20/20, news anchor for Good Morning America, *breast cancer survivor*

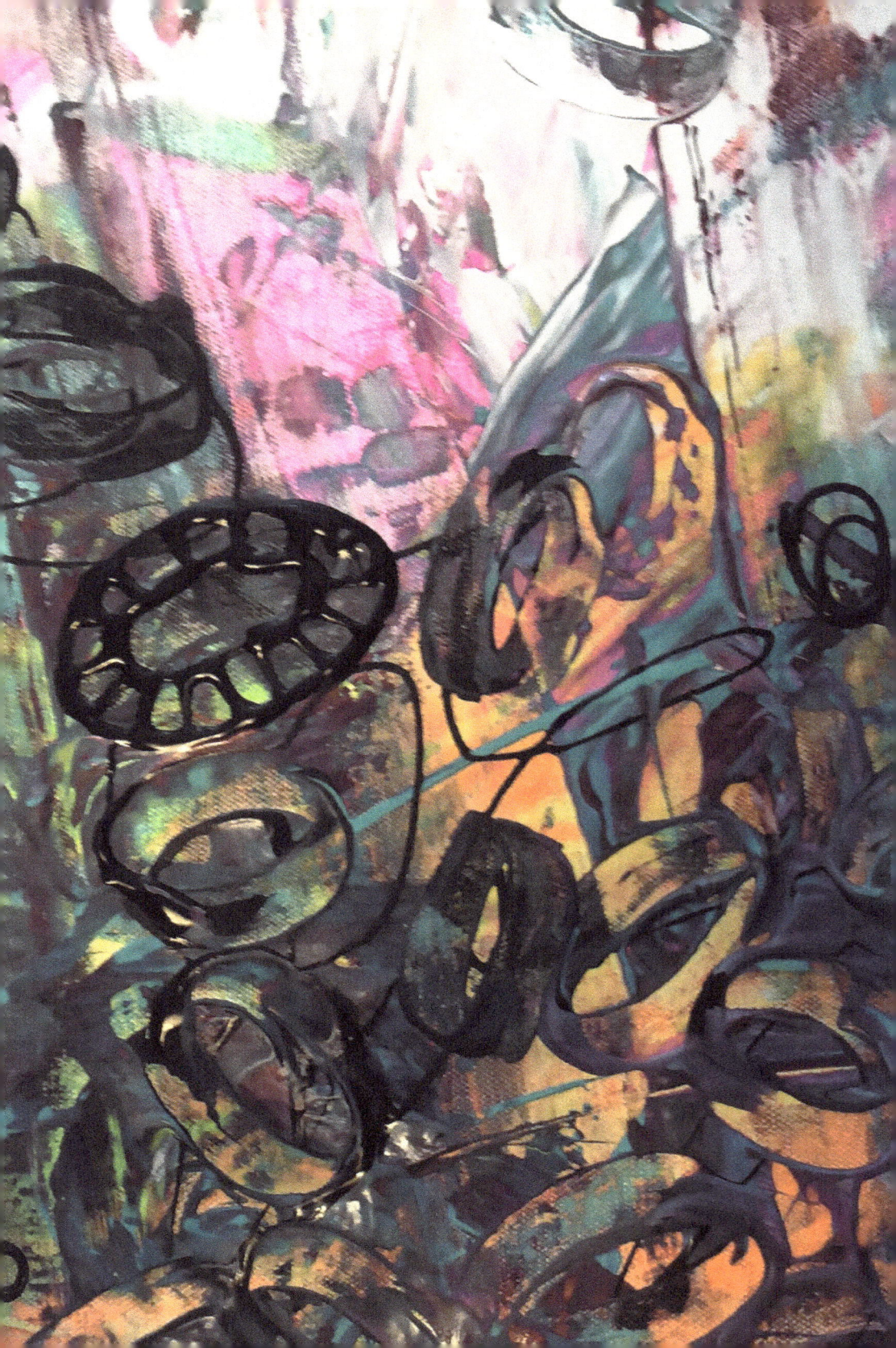

Table of Contents

Darlene   *Linda*
Sue   *Cathy*
Tanya   *Rachel*
Kathy   *Susan*
Rona   *Jen*
Peggy   *Lisa*
Wendy

· · · · · · · · · · · · ·

Introduction

In 1998, my sister, Annette, was diagnosed with lung cancer that metastasized to her brain.

At the time, I was living in Michigan and owned a busy hair salon. One day, out of nowhere, I received a phone call at work from Annette asking if I was able to go shopping for a wig. I was surprised because she had been telling me that she wasn't at all interested in wearing a wig. I couldn't quickly rearrange my schedule, and so I'd told her I'd be happy to join her the next day, but she was determined to go immediately, while she was "feeling it." She insisted on going alone and promised to drop by afterward.

Annette arrived at my salon with a wig that looked nothing like her natural hair. Through her tears she told me how scared she'd felt, and how awful her experience had been—cold, impersonal, and humiliating. My heart was broken. This came at a time when she needed compassion and trust the most.

As I cut and styled the wig to help her look and feel more like herself, the look of relief on her face made my heart sing. It was at that moment that I knew I wanted to help women faced with cancer get through it with dignity.

For many years, I tried to figure out how I could turn my busy hair salon into a calm, private atmosphere for women dealing with cancer, where I could provide products and services that would help make them feel confident and comfortable throughout their treatment.

Finally, fate intervened. I fell in love, got married, and relocated my life. Already a licensed cosmetologist, I furthered my training and became certified as a wig, compression sleeve, and mastectomy fitter. I began

volunteering with the Look Good Feel Better® organization and our local cancer center. I opened Wigs to Wellness & The Mastectomy Boutique. It was a new beginning. And now I'm living my dream—my purpose.

I've worked with thousands of women. Most of them come to me scared, anxious, and overwhelmed. Many times our visits turn into long, intimate conversations about hair loss and all the other "cancer stuff." They ask me why their scalp hurts. They ask me how to cover surgery scars. They ask me what skin creams I recommend. They tell me about a cute little top they found to wear during chemo, a great eyebrow serum, a comfy seat belt cushion; all sorts of practical and fun things they've discovered to feel beautiful, manage their symptoms, and lift their spirits.

They, like many women, spend countless hours searching, trying to understand what's happening to them, and how to deal with their side effects. And many are left more afraid and confused than ever.

It was then I realized there was nothing I could give them or nowhere to point them that would provide all this information in one place. And so, *Healing Pretty* was born. I compiled my years of training and experience, added wisdom from women who've been there, and supplemented it with secondary, research-based resources from medical professionals to create a reliable and comprehensive, head-to-toe guide for women with cancer.

I published the first edition in 2016 and received a wonderful response—not only locally—but from people across Canada and the United States, who ordered copies and provided heartwarming testimonials. I also received more suggestions and recommendations, and more women wanted to share their stories. I'm happy and honored to publish this second edition of *Healing Pretty*.

During this already stressful and complicated time, my hope is to provide you with the information you need in an uncomplicated way.

The priorities of your medical team are to move quickly and efficiently with a treatment plan so that you can get well. My priority is to keep you feeling comfortable and confident along the way.

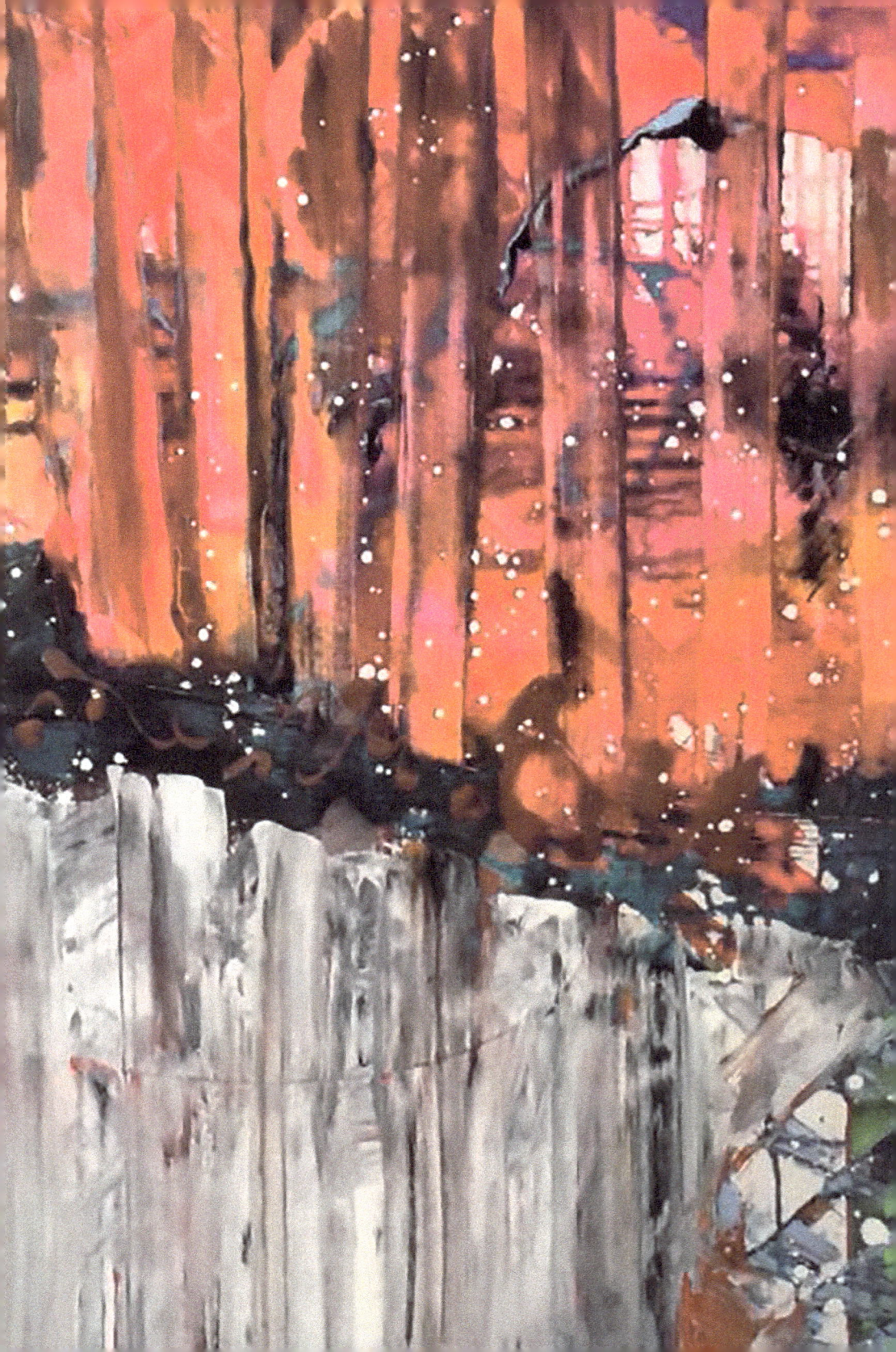

. . . .

Acknowledgments

Cathy Mombourquette: Thank you for being my companion along this journey, and for your personal and professional guidance. You have been there from the very first day that I had the vision of writing *Healing Pretty*. You have gone above and beyond, and I could not have done this without you.

Joe Pizzuti, my husband and collaborator: Thank you for your patience, support, and input. Our late-night chats in your office always managed to get Cathy and me back on track. Who knew a garage could be so inspiring?

My clients: Thank you for the privilege of allowing me to be part of your lives and for allowing me the honor of passing your wisdom on to others.

Dr. Caroline Hamm, MD, FRCP(C): As a medical oncologist, your expert advice made this revised edition a more professional publication. Thank you.

Marie Prevoo: Thank you for generously allowing me to feature your beautiful artwork throughout *Healing Pretty*.

Chris Edwards & Elaine Weeks, Walkerville Publishing: Thank you for your professional design expertise and your patience and passion in helping us complete this project.

Linda Moroun: Thank you for sharing your experience in operating-room protocol.

Shari Mogg: Thank you for your professional make-up and skin-care tips.

Soul Sisters Annette Apostol, Marcia Bear, Michele Bosse, Trish Brookes, Sonia Coletti, Daniella Czudner, Kelly Davidson, Linda Dettinger, Jen Ellwood, Karin Forshaw, Sandra Kavanagh, Kelly Kime, Deb Kokovai, Darlene Kopacz, Jill Laframboise, Sue Litster, Tanya Marra, Jane McGinnis, Kathy McIntyre, Rona Paquette, Peggy Polewski, Linda Santos, Cathy Sebben, Sheila Smith, Rachel Spadotto, Linda Symonds, Susan Szucs, Jen Teti, Lisa Thompson: Thank you for sharing your personal stories and words of wisdom.

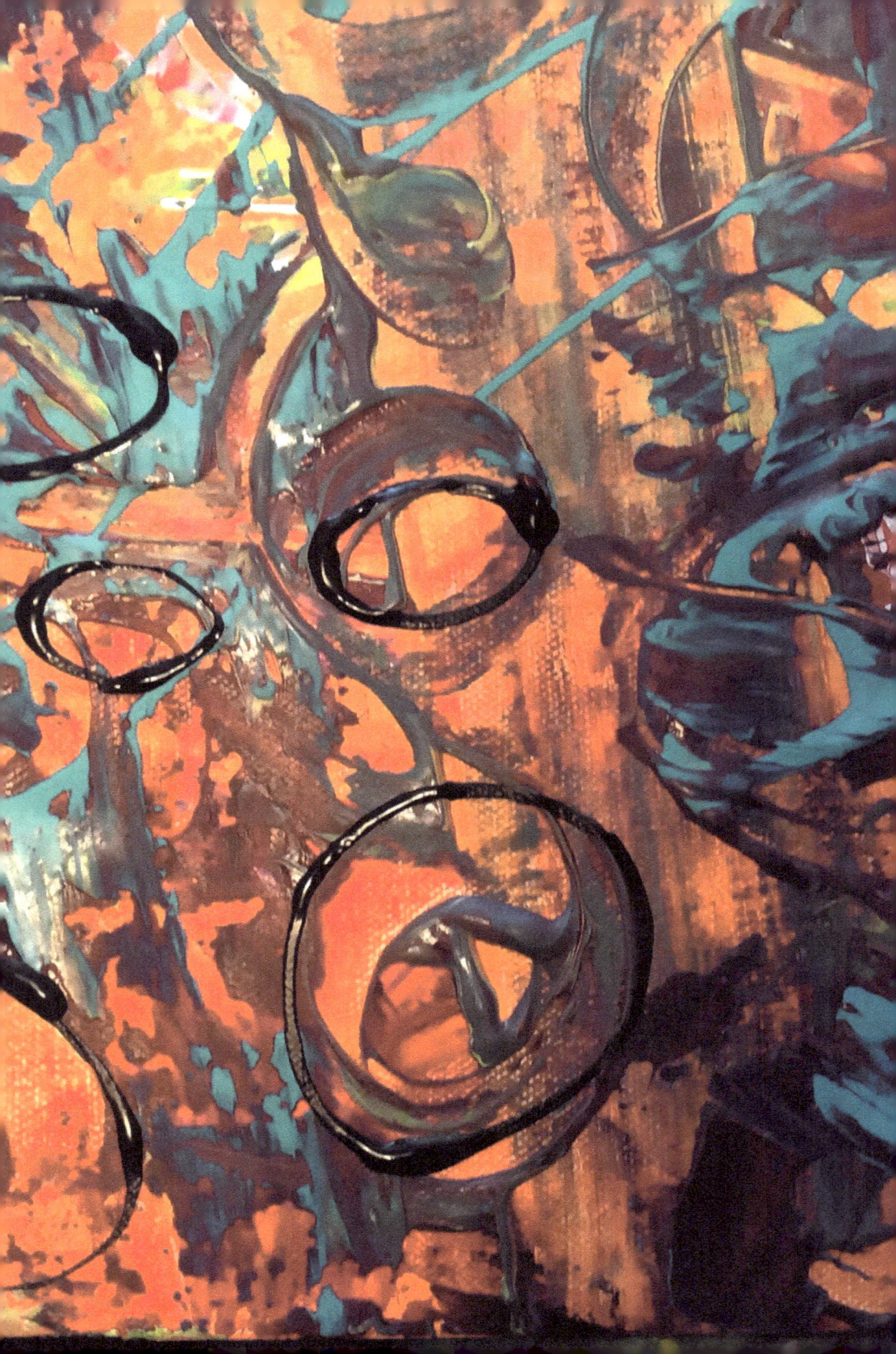

"I've learned to make fearless choices. You come up against stuff now and you're like, All right! Just do it!"

—Melissa Etheridge, singer-songwriter, guitarist, activist, author, breast cancer survivor

. . . .

1
Plan for What You Can

Before treatment begins

From the moment you hear "You have cancer," you will be bombarded with appointments, paperwork, tests, blood work, treatment plans, and more.

Planning is one of the best things you can do for yourself.

Being prepared will help ease your anxiety and let you focus on the road ahead. Here are some recommendations to consider before you begin treatment. Some apply specifically to chemotherapy, and others to treatment in general.

Planning Checklist

- Have your teeth cleaned along with any necessary dental work completed, as your mouth contains bacteria, which could get into your bloodstream and cause infection. With a weakened immune system, you don't want to risk this. Also, you should not have any dental work performed during treatment, unless it's urgent and can't wait.
- Have all routine medical procedures done, such as a Pap smear, eye exam, angiograms, etc.

- If you will be having a mastectomy or lumpectomy, purchase a post-surgical healing bra (see Chapter 8), and be sure to bring it with you to surgery. If you are having reconstruction, ask your surgeon if you'll need a compression bra.
- If possible, shop for a wig *before* treatment if told you will likely lose your hair.
- Clean your home and get organized. The less you must do while in treatment, the better.
- Stock up on disinfectants and cleaning products for yourself and your family, because while in treatment, you'll need to keep the bathrooms in your home exceptionally clean, particularly during chemo. When you begin chemo, always flush twice, as urine can contain traces of chemo and could expose other people.
- Prepare foods and freeze them to make meal planning easier.
- Try to tie up loose ends at work and take care of things at home, like paying bills. These are things you shouldn't have to think about while in treatment.
- Arrange childcare.
- Make sure you own some comfortable and functional clothes for chemo and radiation (see Chapter 8 for great ideas).
- Plan transportation to and from treatment.
- Read *Healing Pretty*.

And from all the stories I've heard from women who've been down your path, it's so important that you look and feel like your normal self as much as possible. It is my hope that the ideas and resources in *Healing Pretty* will help you do just that.

"It's a life-changing thing to be in a position of needing help and being so lucky as to get it. And to feel like that's okay. You can't just take care of everybody else all the time."

—Maura Tierney, actress, breast cancer survivor

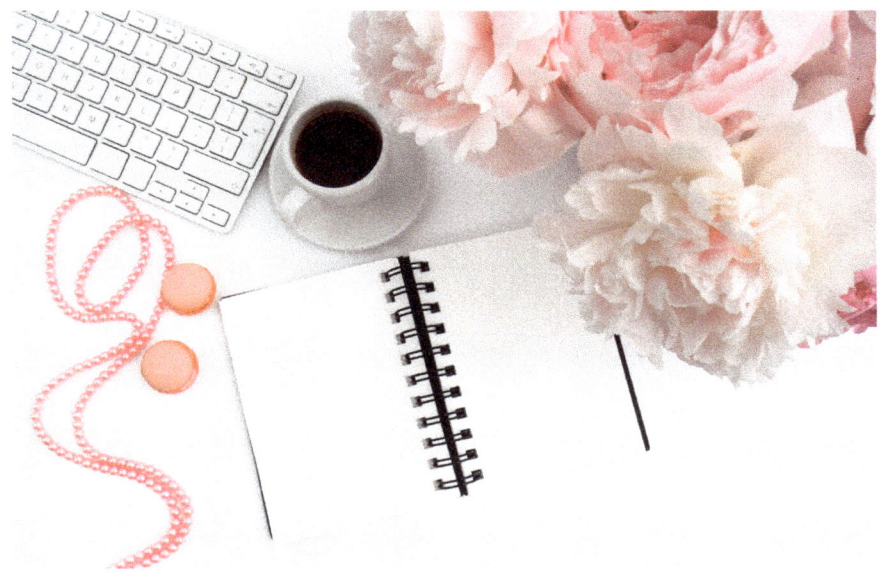

Financial Resources

There are many programs available to help with the cost of some of the products mentioned in *Healing Pretty*. As part of your planning and preparation, be sure to explore:

- Patient-assistance programs and/or financial aid offered at your cancer treatment center.
- Your local Cancer Society branch. Some provide wigs, head-wear, prostheses, and bras.
- Your private healthcare plan.
- Government-sponsored programs.

Fertility Preservation

Many cancer treatments—including chemotherapy, radiation therapy, and surgery—affect fertility and can be permanent or temporary. Therefore, it's very important to talk to your health care team before treatment begins. The following has been adapted from Cancer.net.

There are several ways to preserve fertility:

- **Embryo freezing**: Also called in vitro fertilization; this is where a woman takes fertility drugs for approximately two weeks, then has her eggs collected by a member of her health care team. They are fertilized by sperm in a laboratory and the resulting embryos are frozen until later.

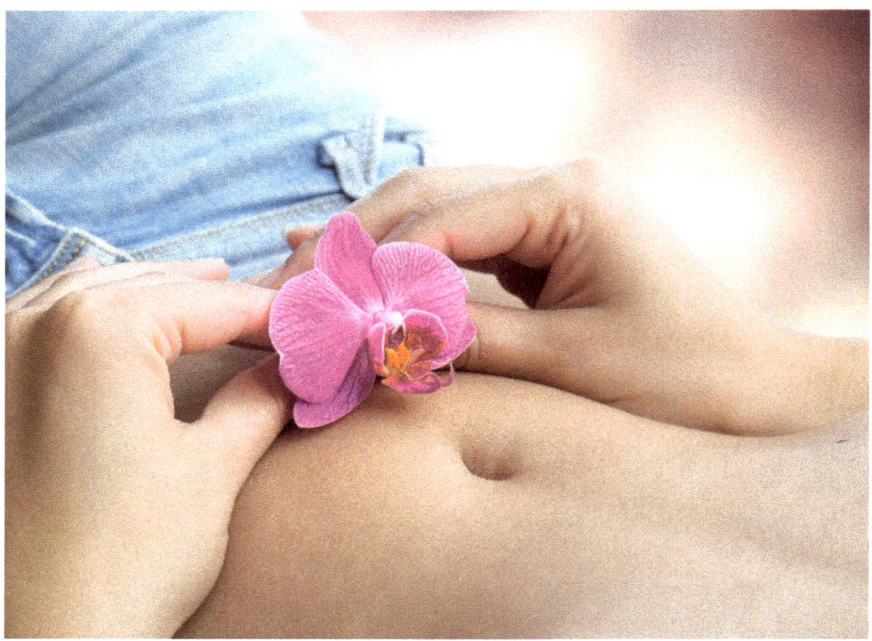

- **Oocyte freezing**: This is similar to embryo freezing, however the eggs are frozen without being fertilized by sperm.
- **Fertility-preserving surgery**: Some types of cervical or ovarian surgery can preserve fertility. For cervical cancer, sometimes surgeons can remove the cervix while keeping the uterus, which allows a woman to deliver by C-section. For ovarian surgery, sometimes surgeons can remove only one ovary, which preserves the healthy ovary for reproduction and prevents early menopause.
- **Radiation therapy that protects the ovaries**: Some women may receive radiation to only one ovary. Another option is

called oophoropexy where the surgeon removes one or both ovaries, then puts them back in place after treatment.

- **Ovarian suppression:** Involves taking hormones that suppress ovarian function, which may protect eggs from treatment.
- **Ovarian tissue preservation**: Involves surgically removing and freezing ovarian tissue, and then the surgeon transplants the tissue after treatment.

There are many factors that affect whether these options are appropriate, such as the type and stage of your cancer, your age, and other factors such as whether the cost is covered by health care plans. These are all important things to discuss with your care team, and as soon as possible before treatment begins.

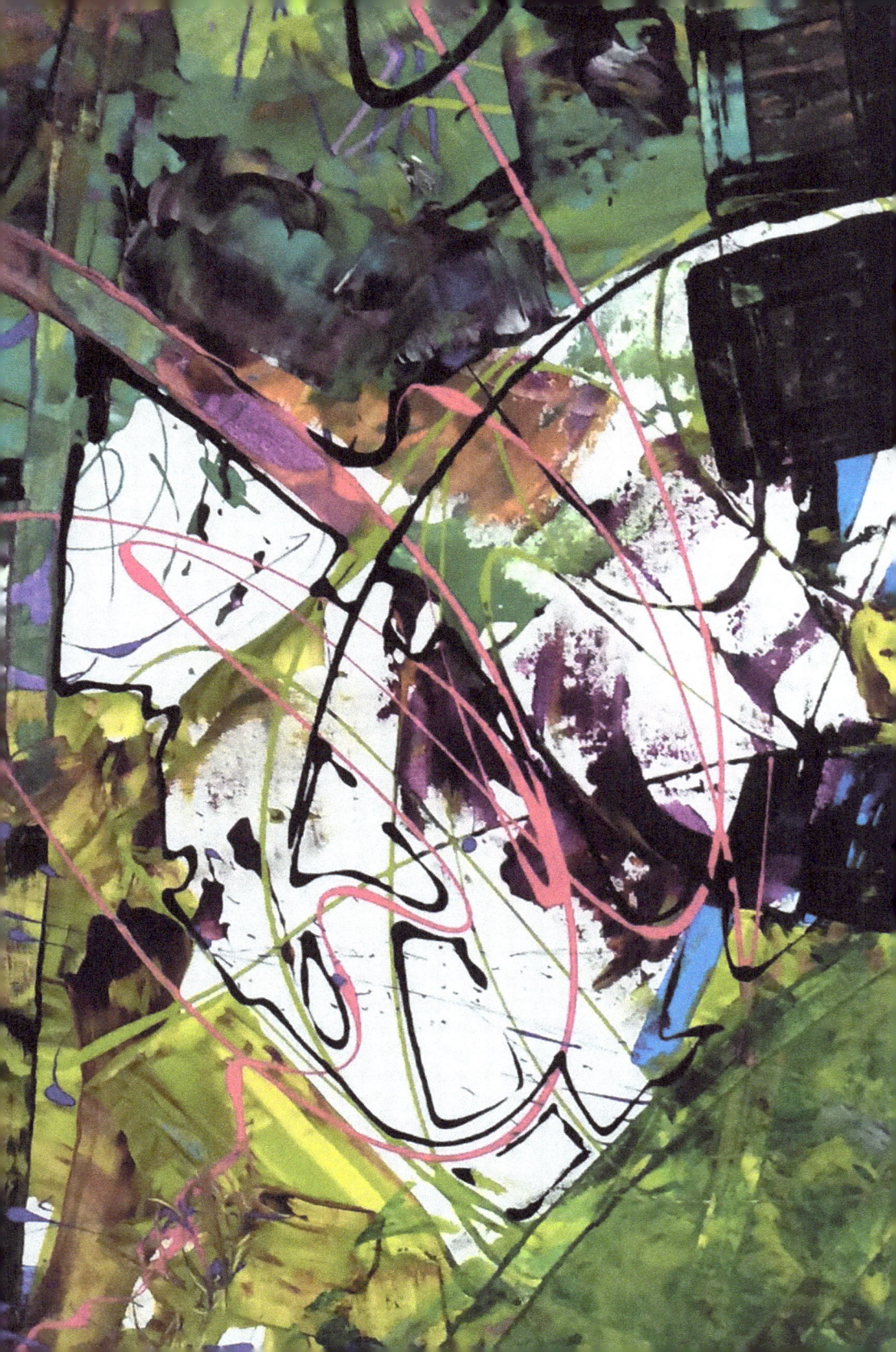

*"Keep your sunny side up,
keep yourself beautiful, and
indulge yourself!"*

—*Betsey Johnson, fashion designer,
breast cancer survivor*

· · · · · · · · · · · · ·

2
Heads Up

Helping you through hair loss

HAIR LOSS

Most women have told me that, second to the initial diagnosis of cancer, the thought of losing their hair is the most devastating.

In the grand scheme of things, achieving optimal health is the primary concern—but we can feel good about our appearance at the same time.

In an ideal world, our hair would have nothing to do with how we feel about ourselves. But for most of us, it plays a significant role in our external identity and influences how we feel. My mother once said, "You can put a million-dollar gown on a woman, but if her hair is not right, the gown means nothing." I admit there is some truth to that. For me, seeing a bald woman walk into a room rocking an evening gown is nothing short of breathtaking, but for most of us, we need our hair to help us feel beautiful.

I'm not going to sugarcoat this process because I know from experience that's not what you want. My goal is to prepare you, preferably before you begin any treatment.

What to Expect

When you receive a treatment plan, talk to your health-care professional about whether it's likely you'll lose your hair. Hair loss, also called alopecia, may be a side effect of chemotherapy, targeted therapy, radiation therapy, or stem cell transplants. These treatments can cause hair loss by harming the cells that help hair grow. You may experience hair loss on other parts of your body as well, such as your eyebrows, eyelashes, legs, arms, underarms, and pubic area. Radiation therapy only affects the hair found where the radiation is directed. And not all chemotherapy causes hair loss. The good news: Most of the time, your hair will grow back.

My advice is to be prepared before any hair loss begins. I recommend shopping for a wig as soon as you're told you'll likely lose your hair.

If you have healthcare coverage, make sure you ask if you're covered for a wig. If so, ask specific questions, such as how many wigs you're permitted and how often you can buy one. Be sure to get a dollar value so that you'll know how much you can spend. You will likely need a prescription from your oncologist to be covered.

Most women will start to lose their hair shortly after their first treatment, a few strands at a time. Now is when you should try your best to come to terms with the process and prepare yourself for the next phase. Again, this will be a much easier course of action if you have already shopped for your wig and/or head coverings.

Shortly after your second treatment, particularly with a breast-cancer diagnosis, your hair will come out rapidly and, in most cases, by the handful. If you choose to let this process run its course, it could be very traumatic for you. Loose hair gets tangled in hair that has yet to fall out and could become a matted mess. Not only is it shocking to find hair on pillows, clothes, in the sink, in your food, and so on, it can also be physically painful. Some women have described it as a throbbing, flu-like feeling in one's head. Most often, that feeling goes away soon after the hair has been shaved.

Rachel's Story

I was diagnosed at age 39 with triple-negative breast cancer. It was a rollercoaster ride the first few weeks; one day I would say, "I've got this!" and the next would be results that changed my journey. After a battery of tests, I received some promising news; the cancer was localized and nowhere else. I had won the first battle but still had the war ahead of me. Ultimately, I knew one thing—if I wanted to beat this, I would have to fight, and to fight, I would need to be strong, to be positive, and to stay true to myself.

I have four children aged 8–14 years old, and telling them was the most difficult part; it broke my heart to see them so hurt. I tried to stay off the Internet—it is a terribly scary place.

About two weeks after my official diagnosis, on my 40th birthday, I had to have a clip-placement procedure and a mammogram. A friend of mine had purchased heart-shaped nipple pasties for me to wear to one of my appointments because she knew it would make me laugh, so I picked my birthday! The radiologist, doctor, and three technicians all had a nice chuckle that day, which lifted my spirits. They told me I had the right kind of attitude that will help to get me through this!

Chemo was up next. I had to undergo chemo first since the breast cancer I had was aggressive and could spread. It was nothing like I expected, like all the stuff you see on TV. They told me that medicine today has come so far. By the end of the treatment, I felt tired and weak with a headache and sinus trouble, but it wasn't too bad, in my opinion (but again, it was only one treatment, so I'm not really an expert).

My next hurdle was the loss of my hair. I brought my 13-year-old daughter with me to choose a wig at Jackie's boutique. I felt empowered by doing this before I lost my hair. We chose it together—it was a nice bonding time for us. Jackie shaved my head during our photo shoot, and I was oddly excited. It was a way of taking control and turning my journey into inspiration for others. I am only at the beginning of my battle, but with all of the amazing people in my life and the support I have received, I'm confident in saying, "We've got this!"—I, my army of friends, my family, and my new Soul Sisters!

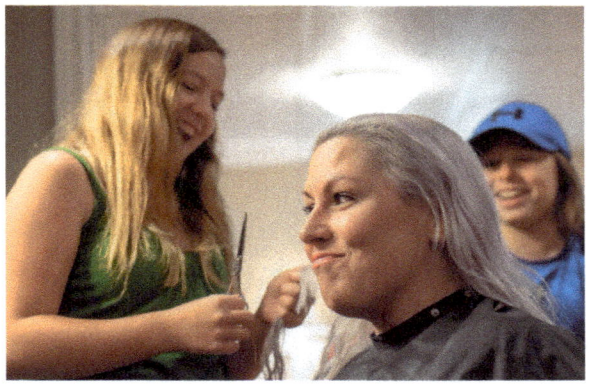

Rachel's daughter Abriana starts with the first cut

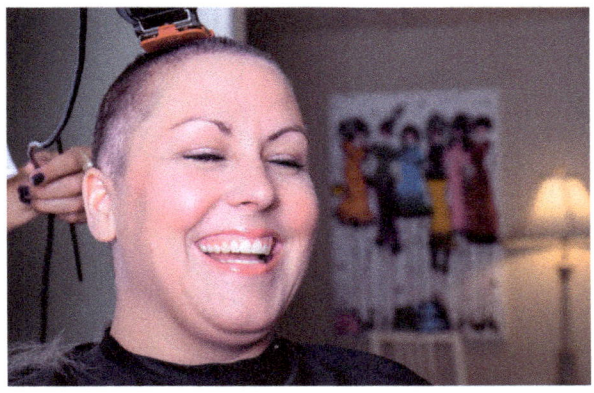

Rachel getting her head shaved

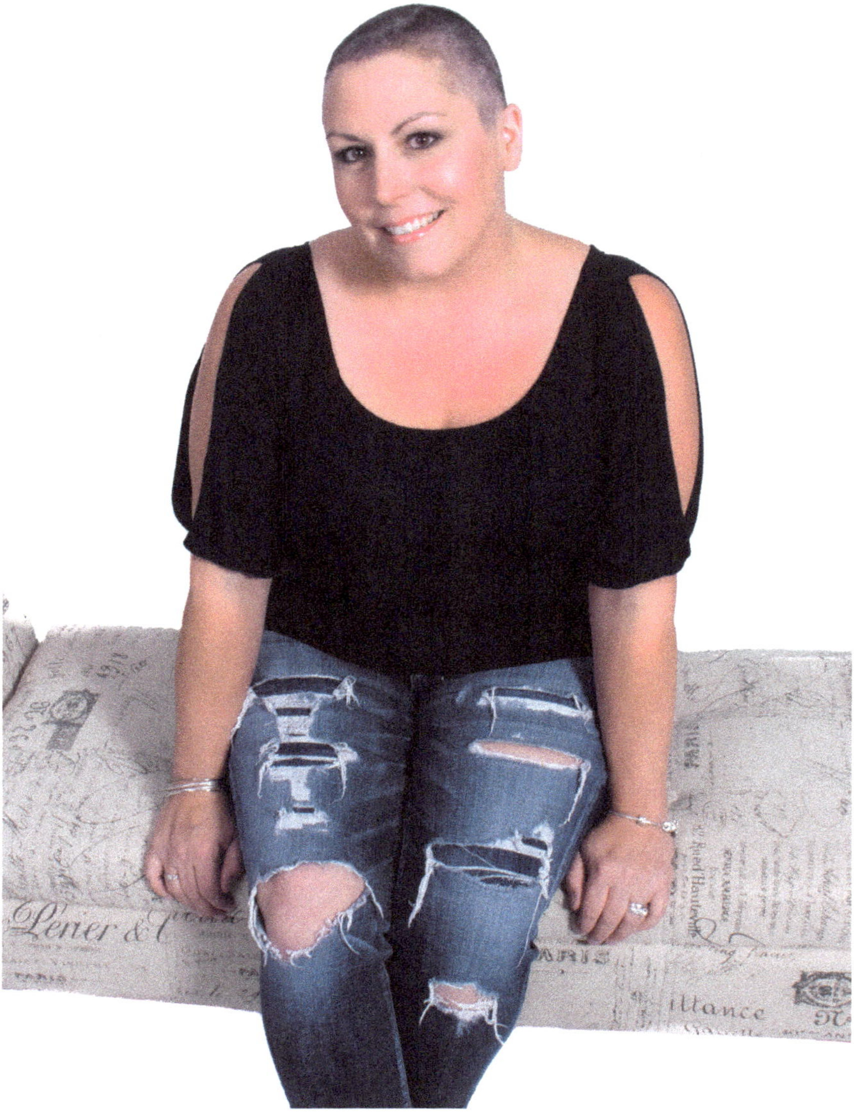

Rachel, bald and beautiful

While your hair is thinning, take care to wash your head and remaining strands no more than twice a week so as not to strip your scalp of nourishing oils. Use gentle shampoos and conditioners without fragrance or dyes, as they are the least irritating.

Taking Control

Taking control of hair loss by opting to shave your head can be incredibly empowering. I recommend a number-one clipper guard, which will give you a close shave without the risk of getting cut. Open wounds could leave you vulnerable to infection, so always take sanitary precautions and sterilize everything before use.

Keep in mind, everyone handles this process differently. Some women prefer to get a few haircuts first, especially if their hair is long. I've seen women get two or three cuts, working their way to a pixie-cut, even if only for one day, before gathering the nerve to shave it. I've seen some women embrace it so completely as to have head-shaving parties with supportive family and friends. I've also seen women hold on to the last ten hairs on their head. There is no right or wrong way to manage hair loss. Whichever way you choose is normal. My goal is to help you feel as comfortable as possible with the process.

For you to come to terms with losing your hair, you can take comfort in knowing there is a huge selection of wigs out there, as well as beautiful headwear to help you look great.

Finding a Wig Salon

Find a reputable wig salon in your area. A personal recommendation is always best, but not always possible. Your treatment center will likely provide you with local resources, and in some cases, they may have a wig boutique on location.

The perfect salon should be able to serve anyone, regardless of race, ethnicity, or religious beliefs. It's a good idea to call ahead and make sure they are equipped to meet your specific needs. They should have a private room for this personal and sensitive visit and a licensed stylist on hand. Not only could this person educate you on different types of wigs and offer guidance as to what would best suit you and your lifestyle, they could also customize the wig by cutting and layering it to help you achieve your desired look and make it your own.

I don't recommend online shopping for your first wig. The expertise, personal touch, and hands-on experience of a wig salon are well worth the extra dollars.

Choosing a Wig

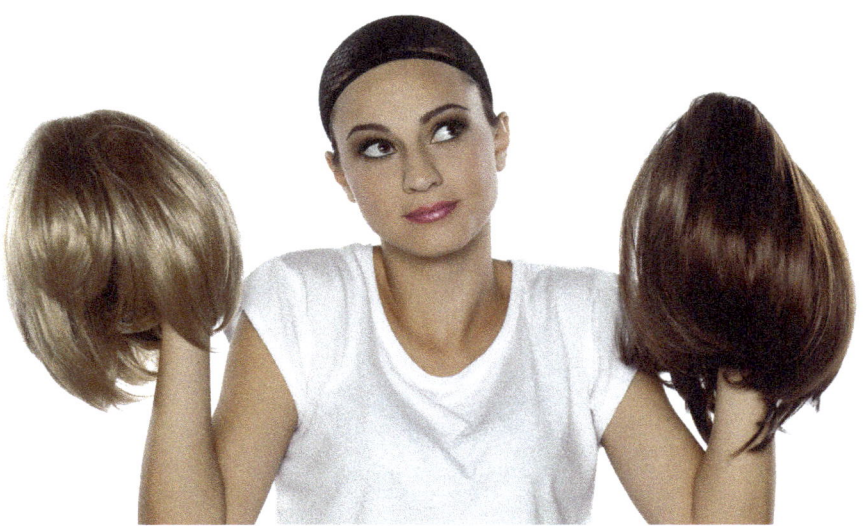

When shopping for a wig, it always helps to bring a trusted friend or family member with you. Their support and opinion will give you the confidence you need to choose the right piece. Also, listen to the advice of the wig expert. They are trained to know what will work best for your lifestyle, and they will help you choose the right color and style—but ultimately, the deciding factor should be how *you feel* in the wig. I've seen women who want it to look as close to their hairstyle and color as possible, and others who want to do something radically different. It's 100 percent your choice.

It's always nice to have a few wigs on hand. Some women will choose two of the same wig and wear one day-to-day and save the other for special occasions. Others will choose two different styles, just for a change.

For some women, wig shopping can be a relatively quick process, and for others, it can take hours, days, and even weeks of struggling to decide. If you're someone who needs the extra time, don't feel like you are being difficult or unreasonable. Both ways are perfectly normal.

TYPES OF WIGS

There are two types of hair used in wig making: human hair and synthetic hair, each of which have different pros and cons, depending on your look and lifestyle.

I've summarized them here, and have included some of my favorite brands.

Human Hair

The most expensive wigs are made from human hair. The advantages are their natural look and feel, as well as the styling options. You can use flat irons, curling irons, and blow dryers on a human hair wig, so you can choose the style you prefer or whichever style you're regularly accustomed to.

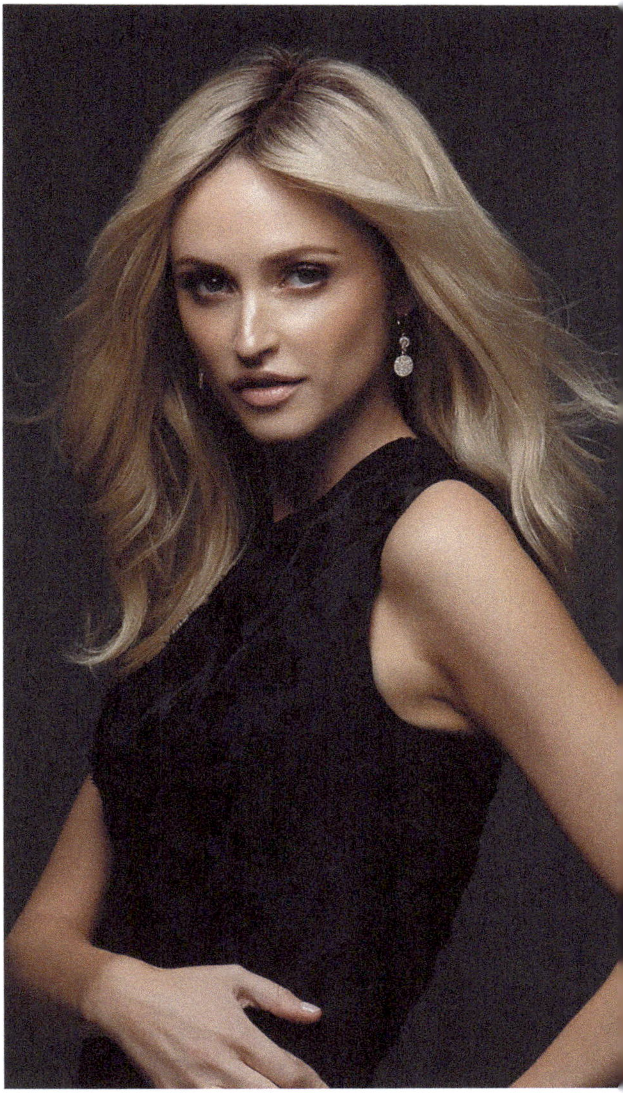

Human Hair Wig by Jon Renau

There are many origins of hair used in human hair wigs, including East India, Brazil, Peru, and Europe, but whichever type you buy, I recommend a Remy processed wig. They are chemically treated to create particular colors and textures, but the cuticles of the hair remain intact. This leads to fewer tangles and a silkier look. You should use human-hair wig shampoo and other specialized products from the boutique where you purchased your wig.

There is more upkeep with this type of wig—for example, your curls will fall with humidity, just like your real hair. So be prepared for a little more maintenance.

Synthetic Hair

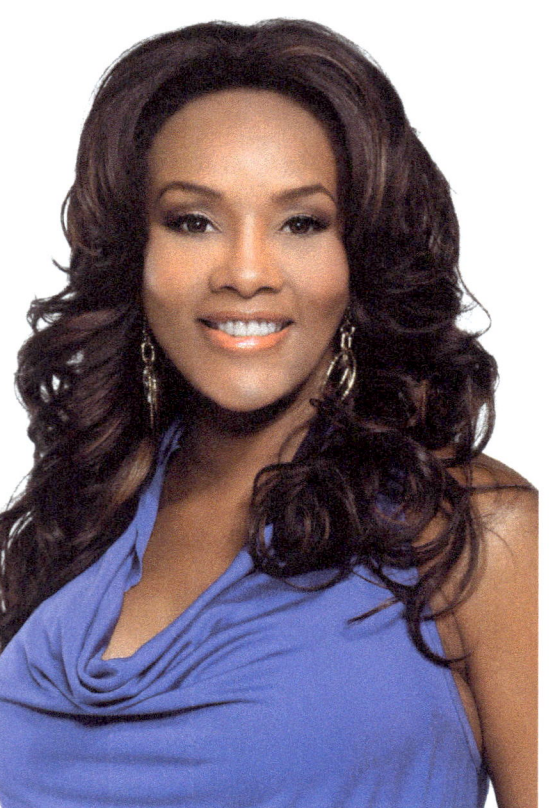

These are the most affordable and the easiest to maintain. And nowadays, they are quite beautiful. Two of my favorite brands are Envy Wigs and Jon Renau.

The downsides to synthetic wigs are their lack of style versatility and low heat tolerance. You can ruin your wig in a flash just by opening the oven door.

Heat-defiant fiber is another type of synthetic fiber that allows you to apply some low-temperature heating implements to it, such as flat irons and blow dryers. I recommend the Jon Renau brand.

Synthetic Wig by Vivica Fox

Personally, though, I'm not crazy about heat-defiant synthetic wigs. They don't curl as well as human hair or human hair/synthetic blend, and you need to be very careful about how much heat you apply. My opinion: If you like the style, go for it, but exercise caution if you intend to use a curling or flat iron on a heat-defiant synthetic wig.

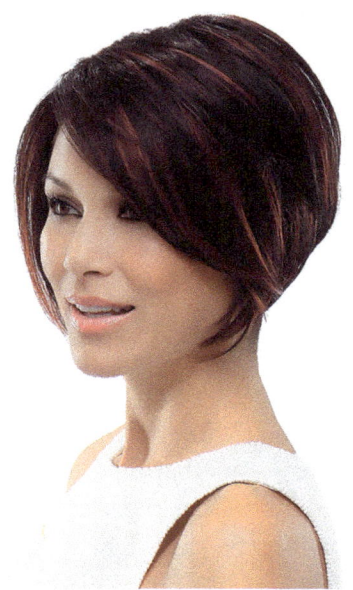

Heat Defiant Wig by Jon Renau

Human Hair/Synthetic Blend

The second most-expensive option is a wig made with a human hair/synthetic blend. I love these wigs. They have the same advantages as a human hair wig, but without the cost. You can use all your heating implements, and with the human hair/synthetic blend, it won't frizz like human hair. These wigs also require less maintenance.

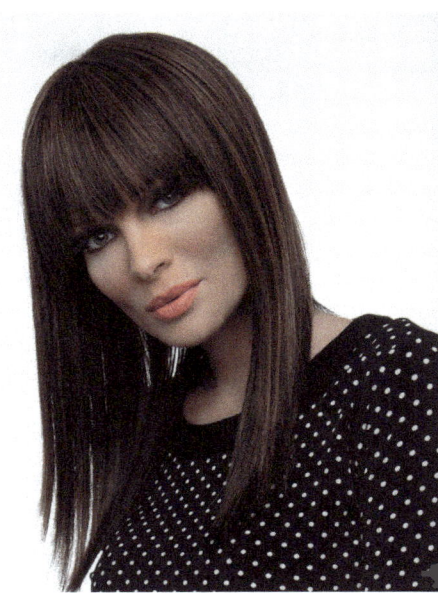

Human Hair/Synthetic Blend Wig by Envy

Custom-Made

Time and cost may both become factors when it comes to custom-made wigs, as the finished product requires a very personalized service, which can take up to ten to twelve weeks. If you decide to go this route, you may want to consider purchasing a less expensive wig while you wait for your custom order to arrive.

Many women have asked if they can use their own hair to make a wig. What they don't realize is that it takes several heads of hair to construct one piece, so this would only be an option if you are willing to combine your hair with that of others. Your wig specialist will advise you on what type of hair is best for you. The better the quality of hair, the costlier the wig will be. Other factors in custom wig construction include size, density, color, curl pattern, and length. There are many types of hair available, from synthetic to virgin (hair that has never been processed).

If you think you may want a custom wig, be sure to find a reputable salon specializing in this process. My recommendation is Truly You Hair Solution Centre, located in Toronto, Ontario, Canada. If you don't live nearby, they offer Skype consultations. See *Appendix B: Resources* for their contact information.

WIG CAP CONSTRUCTION

Now that you know about the different hair options available for your wig, it's important to know about different options for the cap construction of your wig.

If you turn a wig inside out, you'll see the way its cap has been constructed. The terminology below lists the most common features and types of caps. It will give you an idea of what to look for when shopping for your wig. Most of my clients think the longer the hair, the more

expensive the wig. It's not true. The cost of a synthetic wig is in the cap construction. I've broken cap construction into three categories below.

Machine-Made

Every wig company has a different name for this type of cap. To keep it simple, I'll call it "machine-made." These are the least expensive of the synthetics. If you flip the cap inside out, you'll see a cloth material, sometimes with a velvet piece of fabric placed at the front of the wig. You may also see some wefts and solid pieces of material. These wigs are good for someone who prefers a little height, wears a full bang, or is looking for a more mature style.

Monofilament Top

This construction has the same features as a machine-made wig except for a small section on the top of the wig. The cap is made from a sheer material that when placed on your head looks like your natural scalp. It's a terrific feature, especially if you prefer a style that shows any part in your hair.

100% Hand-Tied

This is the costliest type of cap construction. It's entirely hand-tied onto a soft piece of lightweight material that is often made from a soft nylon mesh or silk-like material. It has a very realistic scalp look throughout. Also, the movement of the hair fibers is loose and more flexible, allowing you to change the direction and placement of a hair part and to obtain a natural hair flow.

SPECIAL WIG FEATURES, ACCESSORIES, AND CARE

Lace Front

A piece of lace is sewn in at the front hairline of the wig, with several pieces of hair sewn into it. The lace rests on your hairline and takes on the appearance of hair growing out of your scalp. This is a very nice feature, depending on the wig manufacturer. However if you wear a full bang, the lace front feature isn't necessary.

Ear Tabs

Wigs with ear tabs have flexible materials at the ears that allow you to adjust and contour it to your face. They are also a great tool to let you know that you have your wig on properly. Tip: The tabs should always be parallel to your temple area.

Adjustable Straps

Velcro or adjustable straps can be found at the nape of the wig that allow you to adjust the fit.

Wig Liners

You can wear wig liners under your wig, but this is optional. Some of the reasons you may opt to wear one would be for less perspiration or a better fit. Some women may develop skin irritation from the wig cap, so wearing a wig liner may prevent this. That being said, most of my clients choose not to wear a wig liner.

Here are some types of liners:

> *Nylon:* This is the most economical, but the least comfortable. You'll typically get only a few wears out of them before they tear.

Mesh/Open Top: These are more breathable, allowing for more comfort.

Cotton: These are more expensive and have a heavier construction. They are more comfortable and last much longer than nylon or mesh.

Headline It: This is a name-brand wig liner designed to evaporate sweat. The wicking material pulls sweat to the top layer so that it evaporates continuously, leaving your head cooler in the summer and warmer in the winter. The three-layer moisture system traps oil, salt, and odors, increasing hygiene and comfort.

Wig Sizing

Unfortunately, sizes are limited in the wig industry. Many wigs fall in the average range, unless you choose the custom route. There aren't very many available in petite sizes, and even fewer available in large sizes; however, don't despair if your head isn't an "average" size. There are ways around everything.

The wig should feel comfortable yet secure for a proper fit. When trying it on, move your head in a full circle a few times, making sure the wig stays in place. If it's slightly loose or tight, you can adjust it at the nape of the wig, as mentioned earlier. In most cases, this will be enough to achieve a proper fit. And pay close attention to how it feels around your ears. The ears are a sensitive area, and the wig could become unbearable to wear for more than a few hours if a proper fit around the ears hasn't been adjusted for.

For those of you who can't get a good fit, you can use double-sided wig tape to keep it in place. To use the tape, your head needs to be free of hair. You can also use a gel-like band that you put around your head. I prefer Sure Grip Comfort Wig Liner by BeautiMark. The band is for those who don't have a large occipital bone. (The occipital bone is the

ridge at the back of your head that keeps the wig from sliding up.) I have a small occipital bone, so I tell you this from personal experience.

Wig Maintenance

Wash all wigs in a basin or sink.

If you have a human hair wig, make sure you purchase a human hair wig maintenance kit. And the same goes for human hair/synthetic blend wigs and synthetic wigs—you'll need to buy special wig products for different types of hair. You can buy these at the same place you bought your wig, or they may already be included with your purchase.

You could also purchase a mannequin wig head, along with accompanying clamp stand and T-Pins. These are great to help you easily dry and style your human hair or synthetic blend wig while it remains securely on a table or countertop. These should be available wherever you purchase your wig. There are also many online resources: simply Google 'mannequin wig head'. They are made from different materials. My favorites are made of cork and canvas materials.

Submerge the wig in lukewarm water and add a little shampoo directly to the piece. Washing the inner part of the wig is important as this is where you perspire the most. The hair itself won't get oily without oil glands, so it only needs to be cleaned of outside elements. After washing the wig, rinse it thoroughly and gently squeeze out excess water. You may also gently towel-blot. Always put the wig on a vented stand to dry, as a Styrofoam head could stretch the wig and cause mildew. If you decide on a human hair wig, you may blow-dry it or air-dry it overnight. Always get detailed instructions wherever you purchase your wig. Different companies may advise varied washing techniques.

OTHER ALTERNATIVES

Hats, Scarves, and Wraps

If a wig is not the way you want to go, there are many other options.

If you're a hat person, you can wear one alone or with a partial hair-piece designed to be worn underneath. Hat Magic by Jon Renau is a great option. Hat Magic is a synthetic hairpiece worn over your head with cross-over elasticized bands. Place it on your head and add your favorite hat or scarf for a no-fuss look. Hat Magic features long smooth straight hair that is very natural looking and comes in a variety of shades.

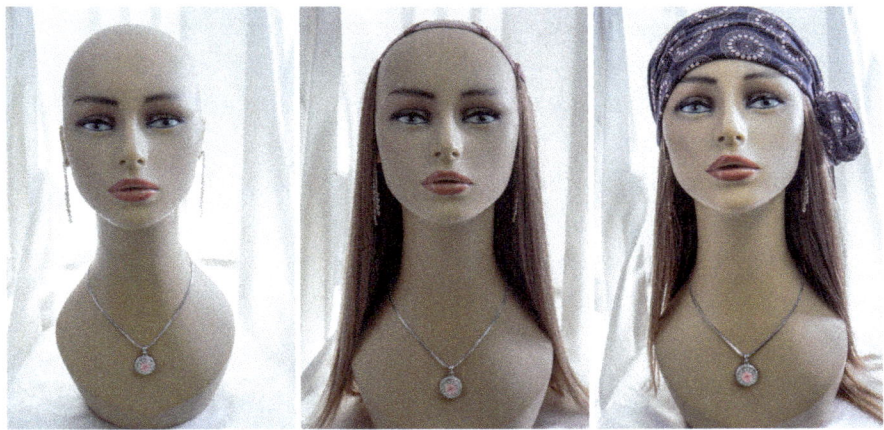

Begin with a bald head   *Add Hat Magic*   *Add your own headwear*

Scarves and wraps are also beautiful. You can add jewels such as brooches or clip earrings to embellish them. If you feel your head is too flat, you can sew in an old shoulder pad to add height; alternatively, you can simply purchase a Tichel Volumizer online (see Appendix B), which is a non-slip, pre-padded cap that gives more height when it is worn beneath one's head wrap.

You likely already have scarves in your wardrobe that you can use. Steer clear of slippery material that could slide off your head, unless you use a soft cap underneath. My favorite material is bamboo, which is very soft and comfortable.

Instead of old-school diagrams of different ways to wrap scarves (which I honestly could never figure out), I suggest using YouTube! YouTube offers a wide variety of scarf wrapping videos by women who are eager to help others like yourself. I've spent hours learning stunning techniques. If you don't have access to a computer, chances are you know somebody who does and would be more than happy to lend you access.

Cold Caps

A cold cap, also known as scalp cooling, is an option worth investigating in to help prevent hair loss. The premise behind cold caps is that freezing the blood vessels in your scalp could help to minimize the amount of chemo that reaches your hair follicles, possibly resulting in better hair retention. The process involves applying a cold gel cap to your head during chemotherapy. As the cap loses its chill, it's replaced with another cold cap, and so on. I don't offer this to my clients because of the relative cost and discomfort involved. However, I believe in the value of research and personal choice.

HAIR RE-GROWTH

In most cases, hair should start to grow back about a month after your last treatment. The average growth rate is approximately a ½ inch to ¾ inch per month. Often, hair will grow back with a slightly different texture than it was before treatment, but given time, it will usually return to its original texture.

There are some chemicals in shampoos and conditioners you might want to consider avoiding. For instance, parabens are chemical substances (a class of preservatives) used not only in shampoos but also in

many cosmetics as well. Parabens have been found in some instances to increase levels of estrogen in the body.

Another chemical often found in shampoos is sulfate, used to attract and break up dirt on the hair and scalp. In some cases, it has been found to be toxic and carcinogenic. It can also cause hair loss and hair thinning because it deteriorates hair follicles and slows hair growth.

Many people are beginning to use paraben-free and sulfate-free products for a healthier scalp and better-conditioned hair.

Hair Coloring

You should wait at least six months to a year before chemically treating your hair, because it will be more fragile. Have a trained professional analyze the texture, elasticity, durability, and porosity first. It's also a good idea to do a test strand before the first coloring.

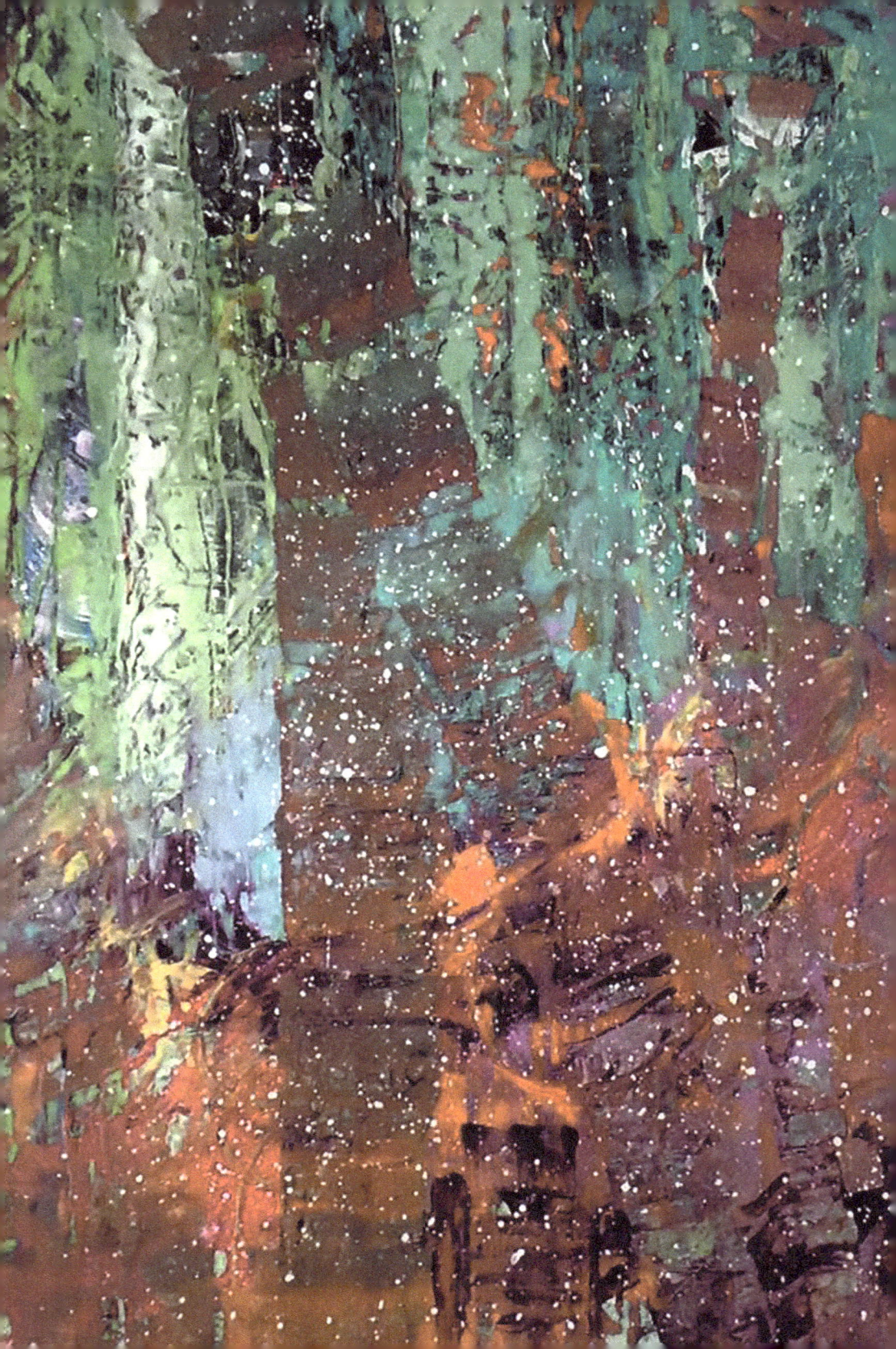

"The only person who can save you is you—that was going to be the thing that informed the rest of my life"

—Sheryl Crow,
singer-songwriter, actress, author, breast cancer survivor

. . . .

3
Keep It Clean

Tips to prevent infection

Good Hygiene Habits

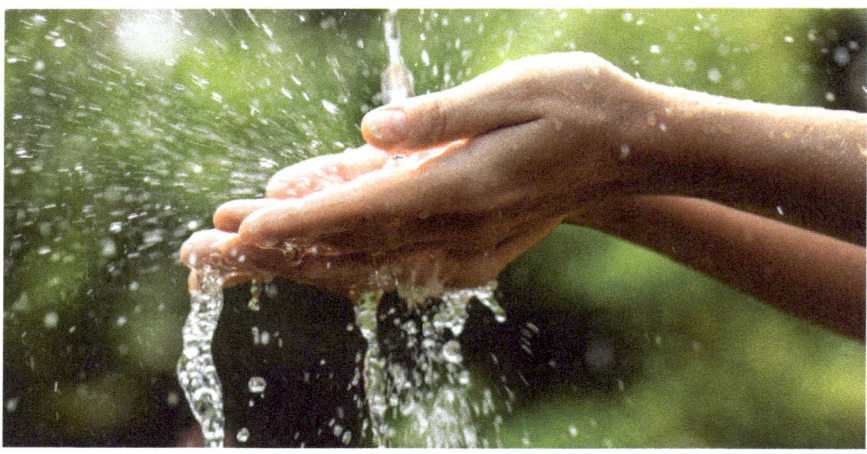

Cancer and cancer treatments can weaken your immune system, making it more difficult for your body to protect itself against germs. It's crucial to do everything you can to avoid infection. Most of the time we don't realize that the things we do on a daily basis can be harmful to us if our immune system is weakened. The following are some good hygiene habits and helpful tips to protect yourself.

- Make sure all your family and friends are aware that if they're not feeling well, they shouldn't come to visit—even if they have something as minor as the sniffles.
- Wash your hands often, with soap and water. Wash them before you eat and before you touch your eyes, nose, or mouth. Always clean up after you go to the bathroom, sneeze, cough, or blow your nose. Other key times to wash your hands are after you've handled trash, gone to a public place, or touched an animal.
- Don't share things with others, like towels, toothbrushes, food, glasses, utensils, etc.
- Keeping your mouth clean is also very important. Good oral hygiene can help prevent thrush (see Chapter 6) a common side effect of chemo. Also, it's advised to refrain from using toothpicks, as they can irritate your gums. Always use a soft toothbrush and be very gentle when flossing. It's also important to rinse your mouth several times a day.

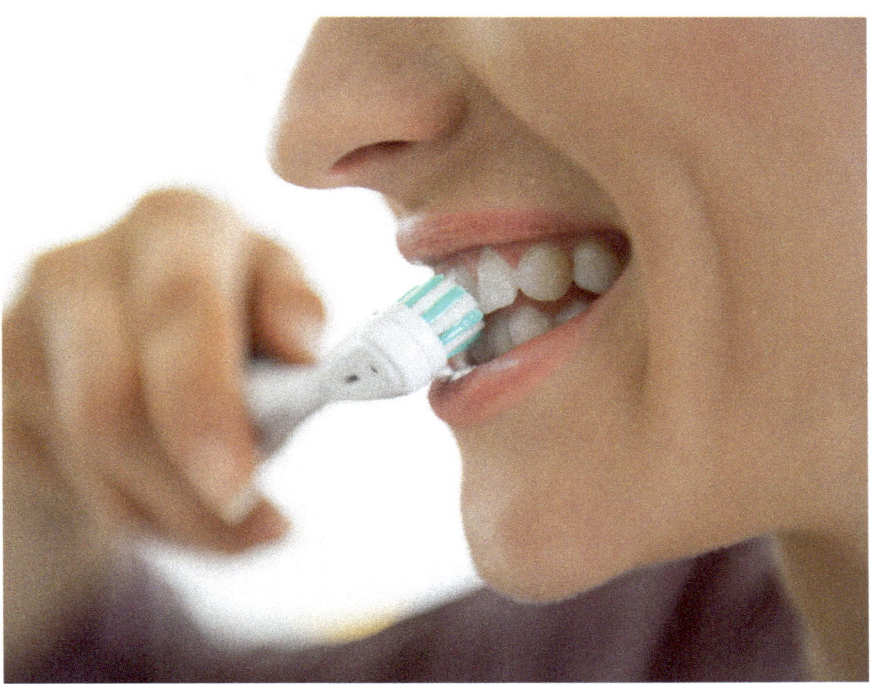

- Always carry non-drying, alcohol-based hand sanitizer with you.
- Try to avoid public places. If you do go out, use cleaning wipes before you touch door handles, elevator buttons, ATM keypads, or any surfaces used by a lot of people.
- Wear a mask when necessary.
- If you develop a rash, try not to scratch.

Grooming Safety

- Be cautious when shaving. Consider using an electric shaver instead of a razor.
- Never use any product past its expiration date.
- Do not share products.
- Never reinsert any cosmetic brush or applicator that has already contacted your skin back into the make-up container.

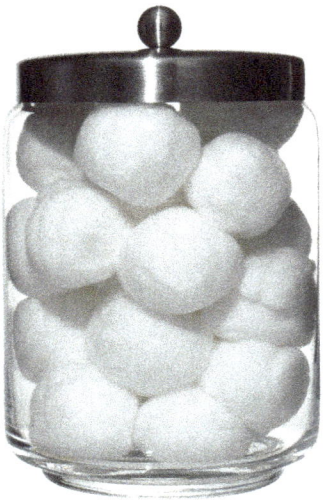

- When applying make-up, always use cotton balls, spatulas, sponges, and disposable mascara wands. You can get these items at a beauty supply store for professionals, many of which are also open to the general public. I prefer buying directly from a beauty supply store when possible, as they are generally of better quality; however, if you don't have one in your area, most dollar stores and drug stores carry these items as well.

- When applying moisturizer or foundation, use a make-up spatula to transfer the product from the container to your wrist, and then apply to your face or body. Pumps are also a great option.

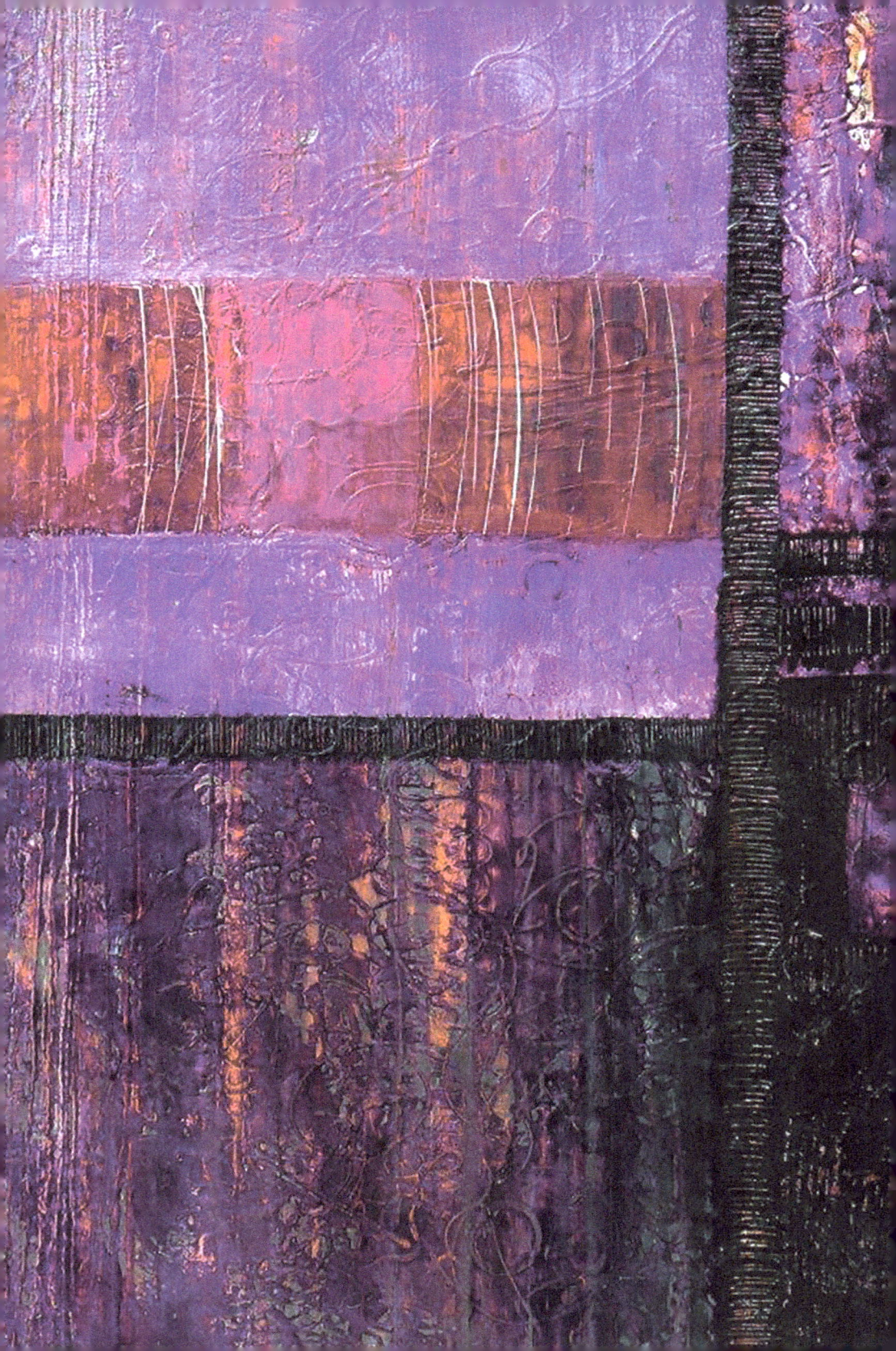

"One important thing is to know you're still the same person during it. You're stripped down, near zero, but it seems that most people come out of it at the other end feeling more like themselves than ever before. I'm more eager than ever to do what I did. I want to do everything."

—Kylie Minogue, singer-songwriter, dancer, actress, author, breast cancer survivor

. . . .

4
Let's Face It

Facial care and make-up tips

Before my sister's diagnosis, she worked for many years as a make-up and skin consultant for Elizabeth Arden in one of Detroit's oldest and largest department stores, J.L. Hudson (now Macy's). I learned many make-up techniques from Annette, but it wasn't until I started volunteering with Cosmetic Alliance Canada's *Look Good Feel Better* program (LGFB) in 2011 that I learned most of what I'll be sharing in this chapter.

Offered in 27 countries, LGFB is a hands-on workshop that educates women with a cancer diagnosis on what could happen to their hair, skin, and nails during treatment. Plus, select locations offer education on the proper fitting for bras and information about post-surgical bras and prostheses. This great program is delivered by qualified volunteers who are trained professionals specializing in hair, skin, make-up, and bras. LGFB also serves as an escape from the overwhelming and seemingly endless onslaught of medical jargon. LGFB is uplifting and, in many cases, a place where women bond and go on to develop close friendships. You'll also receive a complimentary gift bag with brand-name beauty products, from skin care to make-up. This is something you won't want to miss. Ask the staff at your treatment center for registration information, or go to www.lookgoodfeelbetter.org to

find a program near you. They also offer online makeup tutorials and virtual workshops.

Feel More Like You is also a great program, offered at select Walgreens across the United States. Staffed by beauty experts specially trained to manage the esthetic side effects of treatment, their program is free and no appointment is necessary.

In putting together this chapter of indispensable information for optimal skin care and make-up during cancer treatment, I consulted with my close friend and fellow LGFB volunteer, Shari Mogg. Shari is a certified aesthetician and cosmetician who has been working in the industry for over 30 years, helping thousands of women to look and feel their best. She has been volunteering at LGFB for 18 years, often in the role of Team Leader. Here is what Shari would like to share:

SKIN CARE

Cleanse

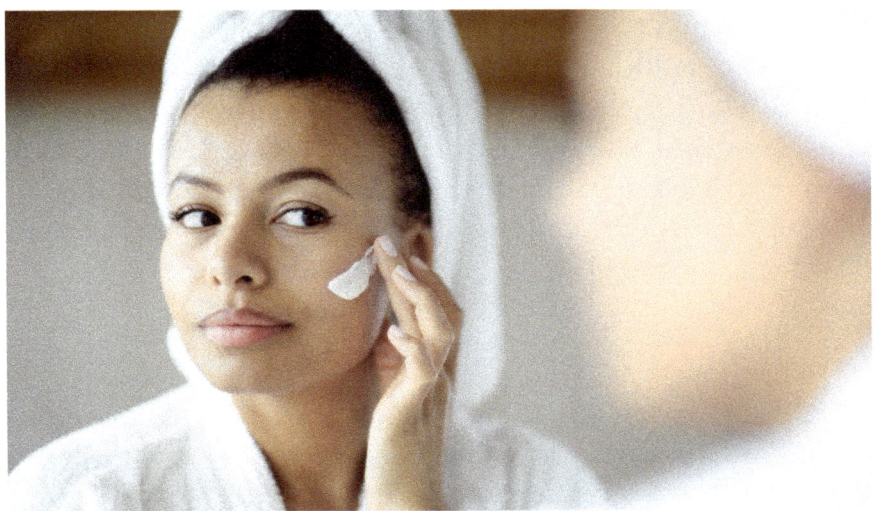

You may continue to use your favorite facial cleanser, as long as it's not too harsh. Make sure the water is never too hot; tepid to warm water is always best. Preferably, though, you should use hypoallergenic and fragrance-free products. This will make it less likely you'll develop sensitivity issues. While there are no guarantees, the gentler you are on your skin, the less likely you'll run into problems.

Tone

You can use your favorite brand of toner, or you can try something as simple as witch hazel. Witch hazel is a natural astringent (be sure to use an alcohol-free brand) and can help control inflammation while soothing skin. It also lessens the appearance of pores and is thought to prevent bacterial growth.

Moisturize

Dehydration is a serious concern for cancer patients because many of the side effects of chemotherapy treatment rob the body of water and electrolytes. Keeping yourself hydrated is of utmost importance. Drink plenty of water and keep yourself moisturized from head to toe. Moisturizer works best when applied to damp skin. Your skin will crave moisture, so don't forget the rest of your body: a good lip balm, cuticle cream or oil, and hand and body lotion should give you some relief from the lack of moisture your skin may be experiencing. Moreover, while dehydrated skin may take on a dull and lifeless appearance, hydrated skin will appear more radiant and supple, and will also feel softer to the touch. If you don't have any hair on your head, you can apply lotion there as well.

Protect

Sunscreen is always important, and especially during treatment. Certain forms of cancer treatments can make people more sensitive to the sun. Use a broad-spectrum SPF 30+. Please be aware that a make-up foundation or moisturizer with SPF is not enough to protect

your face—you still need to apply sunscreen. And don't forget your lips—use a gentle SPF lip balm. For more information about photo-sensitivity and ways to protect yourself, please see Chapter 6.

MAKE-UP

For most of us, putting on make-up is our go-to for feeling pretty. I recommend continuing to use the products you love. However, since your skin is undergoing changes, you may find you'll need some adjustments to your normal make-up routine. Unless it's for a special occasion or you simply prefer a full make-up look, a light and natural look may be the easiest and 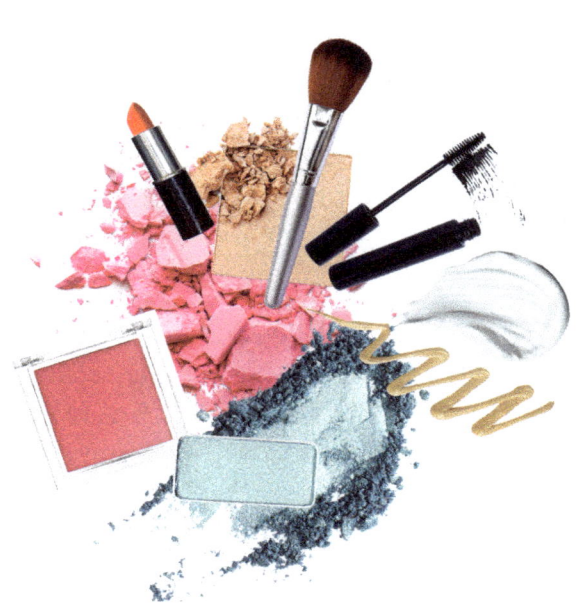 least time-consuming to achieve during your treatment. Here are a few suggestions that may help while you are going through this transition.

But please remember: There is only *one* you! So whatever it is that personally helps you get through this journey is *right*! No one knows your body, your mind, or your spirit better than you. So go with what you feel is true to yourself.

To help avoid infection, be sure to wash your hands before applying makeup. Buy new make-up before starting treatment.

Foundation

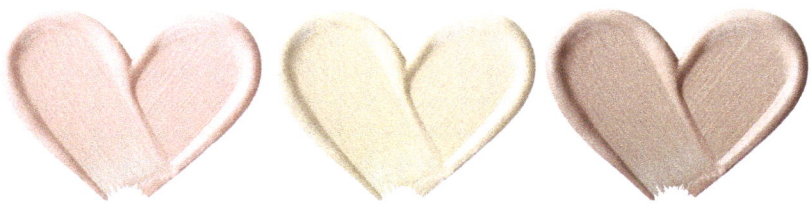

A light beauty balm (BB) cream or color correction (CC) cream may do the trick. Think of these as half foundation and half moisturizer blends. They provide a light to medium coverage, yet they give your skin some of the added moisture it is craving.

Concealer

It's a girl's best friend when it comes to make-up. Concealer is condensed foundation, which is why it covers so well. It's great for dark circles under or around the eye area and covering up redness or sallow skin. These come in many colors and textures, so seek help from your favorite cosmetics store to find the best one for you.

Blush

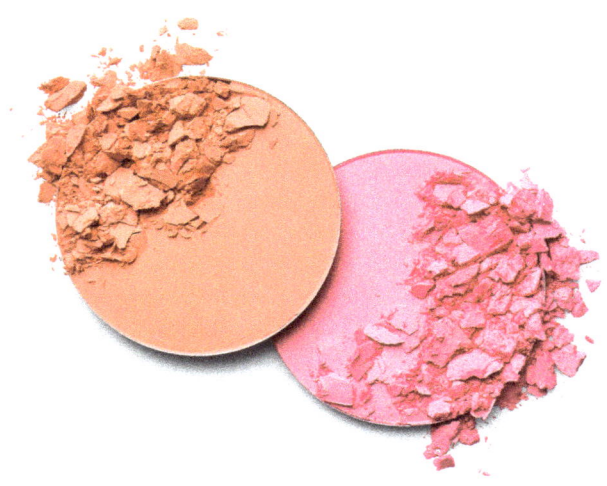

It gives a little glow to the cheek area—who doesn't like a hint of color for a healthy look? Blush comes in the forms of a powder, cream, stick, or pot container. Personal preference will help you decide what works best for you.

Mascara

This is a favorite cosmetic item for many women. Mascara comes in many colors and formulations, and mascara wands come in many textures and style choices—so when you find one that works well for you, keep with it. And to help prevent infection, replace your mascara monthly.

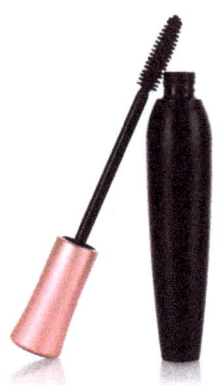

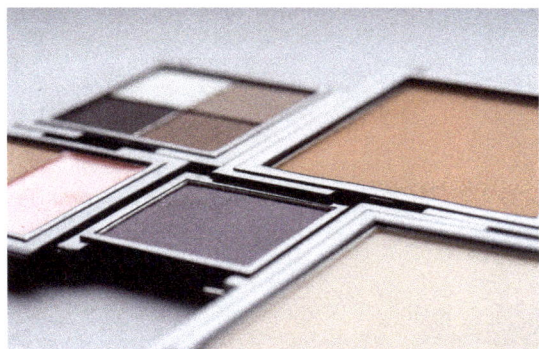

Eyeshadow

This can bring a nice pop of color to the eye area. If your eyes seem to be lacking a bit of luster, a nice light shadow can really open them up.

Eyeliner

This gives the eye a nice wide, bright, and open look. Eyeliners come in many forms, including pencil, liquid, cake form, and more. Your liner should glide on like butter, without pulling or tugging at the skin. Also, if you like to put your liner on the water line (the inner rim of your eyelid), make sure your liner is kohl or khaj, which means it's safe to use in that area. And like mascara, to help avoid infection, replace your eyeliner monthly.

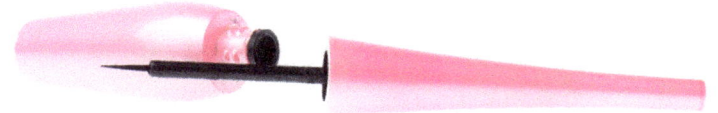

Lipstick

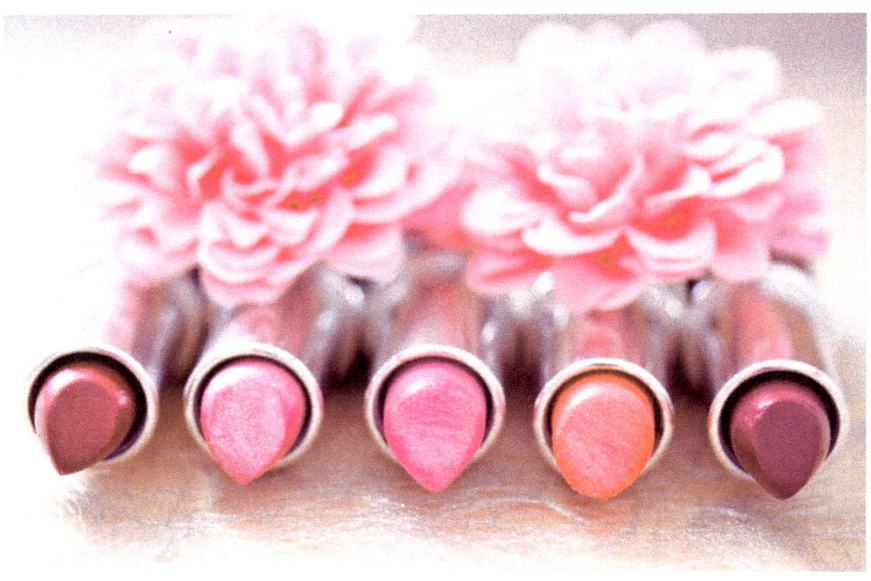

This is the fastest way, by far, to give some color to your face. You may use a lip liner first, if you like to give a bit of definition. If you like shine, there are great lip glosses you can use, or perhaps a tinted balm for moisture and a bit of color. Whatever you choose, have that color be something that makes you smile and *keeps* you smiling!

Here are some other helpful tips for getting through treatment while looking your best. Most of these came from my Wigs to Wellness clients.

EYEBROWS

If you lose your eyebrows or they become sparse, here are some great solutions:

Eyebrow Stencils

You can find eyebrow stencils at most cosmetic counters. Make sure you position the stencil just right; if you stencil the eyebrows too high or too low, this will be a dead giveaway that they're not your own. A great product is SurvivorEyes Brow Styling Kits. Their kit contains 10 brow templates, a dual sided applicator, and a purse-size mirrored compact with powder cosmetics and sealing wax. They're long wearing and smudge proof.

Eyebrow Pencils

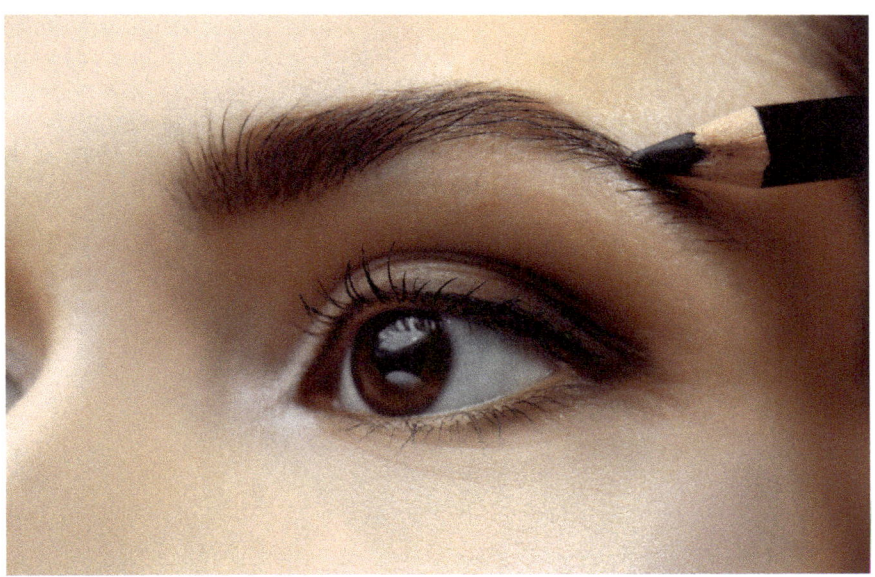

You can find eyebrow pencils everywhere makeup is sold. When using an eyebrow pencil, use quick, short strokes, and never draw a solid line. If you'd like to watch a tutorial, search YouTube for "Look Good Feel Better Brow Tutorial", which does a great job of explaining each step.

Eyebrow Wigs

Eyebrow wigs can be made with synthetic or human hair. Eyebrow wigs affix to your face with a special glue. They come in different shapes, from high arch to a straighter style, and different shades, from dirty blonde to black. Be sure to do a patch test first as you may have a reaction to the glue or the remover.

Here's a great human hair product: Natural Brow Eyebrow Wigs by NaturaLash. The hairs are woven through a semi-transparent backing in beautiful natural eyebrow shapes. They're intended to be applied in the morning and removed in the evening.

Microblading

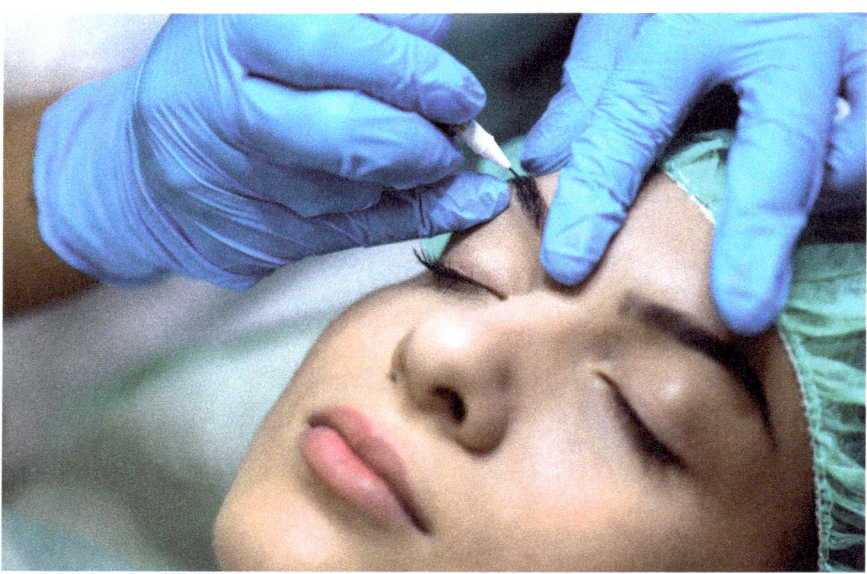

Microblading is a semi-permanent tattoo. It has existed for a long time as a cosmetic procedure and is now being used as a method of brow enhancement. Some women get this done *before* treatment—make sure you're healed before treatment begins. Do not get microblading while in treatment due to the risk of infection. And if you decide to do

this after treatment, you should not be microbladed until six months post-chemo, also due to the risk of infection. Be sure to ask your care team for their recommendation.

If you have a sensitivity to nickel or other metals, you should not use this procedure if traditional tattoo ink is used. There are microblading services that use plant-based materials; seek these out whenever possible. If you are immunosuppressed, microblading is not recommended.

Like anything else, get informed. Make sure you go to a reputable place, and ask for referrals and pictures of their work.

Eyebrow Enhancing Serum

Eyebrow enhancing serum works to help condition and improve the appearance of fuller eyebrows over time. Some formulas include brow enhancing, conditioning, moisturizing, and strengthening ingredients that work together to help improve the overall appearance of eyebrows. Some of my clients have found RapidBrow to be a great product; it's ophthalmologist and dermatologist tested, and fragrance and paraben free. Note that these growth serums aren't effective during treatment, but you can start using them after your last day of chemo.

EYELASHES

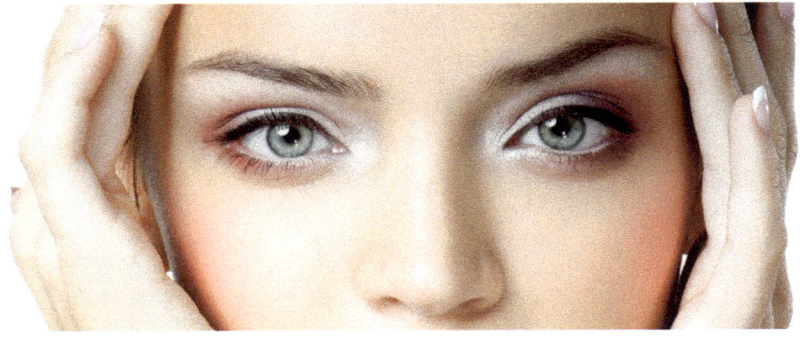

If your eyelashes have become sparse, or you've lost them completely, you can use make-up to create the illusion of having them.

- Cover your upper eyelid with a neutral eyeshadow. Then, using a fine-tipped brush, use a darker color of eye shadow as close to your lash line as possible and apply with short upward strokes. Smudge the shadow a bit to give it a softer look, which will give the illusion of fuller lashes.
- Use the same technique on the lower lash line; however, feather in short, downward strokes.
- Then, using a liner on your lash line, make tiny dots across the lid. This will also give the illusion of fuller eyelashes, but this may take some practice.

Avoid false eyelashes, as there are harsh chemicals in the glue.

Don't get discouraged if your eyelashes fall out after chemo has finished, or if they fall out again after they've started to grow back. Although I've not found any documented proof, I've had some clients share this with me, and I've also read blogs on this topic: In most cases, your lashes will grow back just as full as they were before treatment. For a little boost, you can try eyelash growth serums, such as Latisse, which is a prescription formula, or GRANDLash-MD. Again, these won't be effective until after you're done treatment.

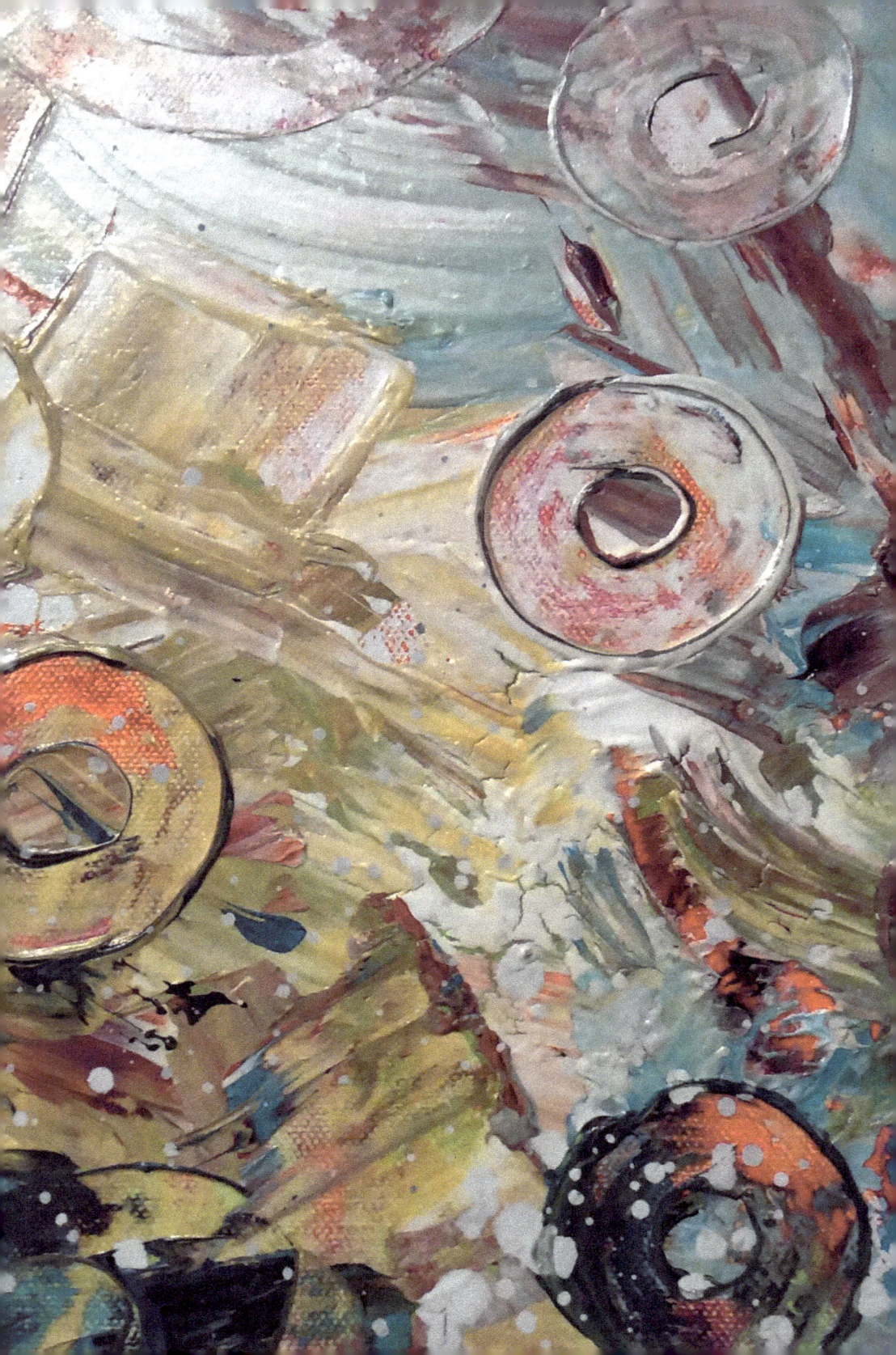

"The art of life is not controlling what happens to us, but using what happens to us."

– Gloria Steinem,
women's rights activist,
author, breast cancer survivor

. . . .

5
You Nailed It

The do's and don'ts of nail care

MANICURES AND PEDICURES

Many of us have become reliant on the convenience and attractiveness of acrylic and gel nails. However, these products can lift, creating an ideal breeding ground for bacteria. Acrylic and gel nails are not recommended while in treatment.

It's also recommended to pay close attention to your nails daily, so it's best not to use polish unless it's clear-coated or sheer. Use nontoxic, water-based lacquer.

Check your nails regularly for color changes, lifting, cracking, or heavy vertical or diagonal lines. These could indicate infection, which should be immediately addressed by your medical team.

If your nails have been damaged, you can help avoid infection by doing a daily antibacterial soak. An easy recipe is to mix equal parts water and distilled white vinegar and soak your nails for 10 to 15 minutes.

You may give yourself a manicure with your own sanitized supplies. You can soak your cuticles and push them back with an orangewood

stick, but abstain from cuticle cutting. If you cut yourself, it can leave you vulnerable to infection. Crystal nail files are preferable not only during treatment but as a lifetime choice. If cared for properly, they can last several years. Another bonus: They can be washed and sanitized.

Personally, I'll never go back to emery boards. The coarse material can damage your natural nail, especially when not used correctly. Be sure to file in one direction. Filing in a back and forth motion can cause splitting and peeling at your nail's edge.

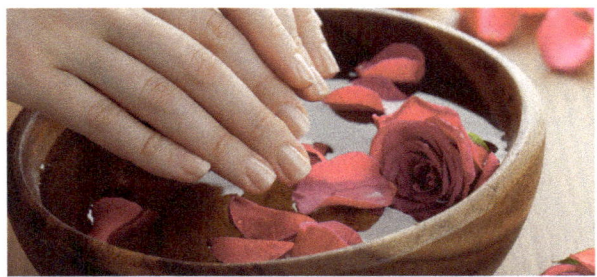

While in treatment, I don't recommend public nail salons. But if you decide to go, be sure to supply them with your own nail-grooming tools. Never share. If you enjoy a pedicure, opt for a stainless steel or glass basin to soak in, versus a basin with a drain which can harbor germs.

Common side effects of treatment include dryness, cracking, and brittleness. Stay moisturized by massaging creams or oils in and around your nail bed.

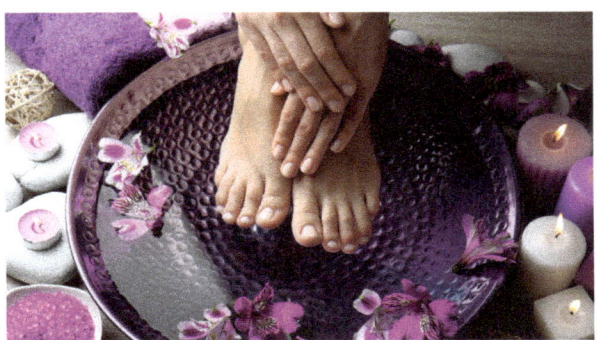

COLD GLOVES AND SOCKS

You may want to consider cold gloves and socks. These are the same concept as the cold cap discussed in Chapter 2. Treatment centers may offer these or you can purchase them online. This method could help prevent nail damage and lifting. Be sure to get your medical team's approval before using this method.

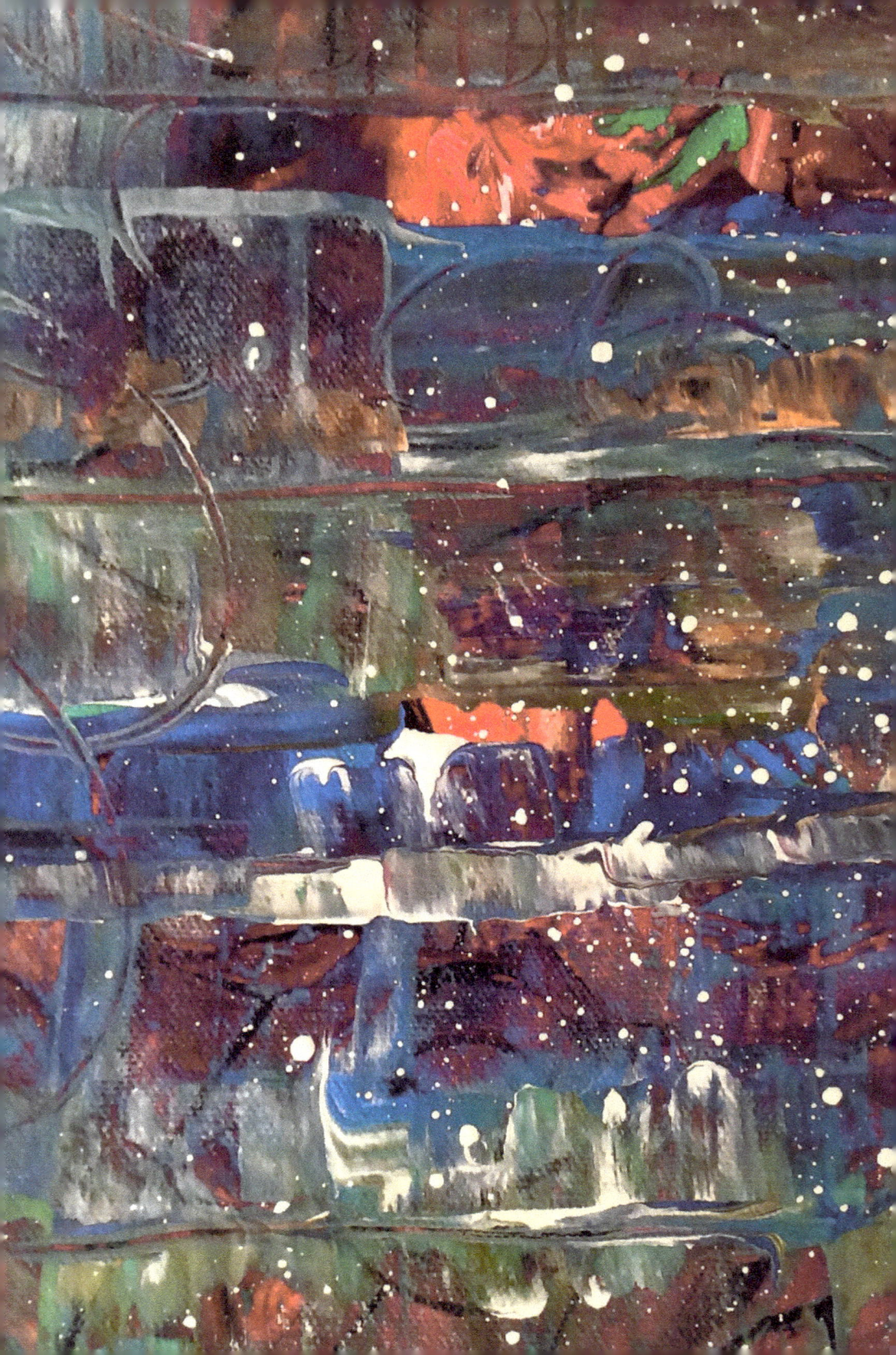

"I just want to show off my scar proudly and not be afraid of it."

—Carly Simon, singer-songwriter, musician, breast cancer survivor

. . . .

6
SOS

Some other side effects

This chapter deals more specifically with our skin and some of the other unpleasant, and sometimes embarrassing, side effects of treatment.

I found that many of my clients were blindsided by some of the unexpected effects, so my hope is that this will help you recognize the early warning signs to help you minimize the problems.

Every side effect is as individual as you are, and they can range from mild to severe. Be aware of any changes and bring them to the attention of your care team; they may prescribe something to help.

Each side effect discussed here is accompanied by recommended solutions. My clients have used most of these products and found them to be effective. Most are available at your local drug stores. There are also organic options. Some of my clients have used products from a local company called Ocean Bottom Soap Company with excellent results, and they ship worldwide. Another great option is Soap Chef (also local), and they give a 10% discount for those going through cancer treatment. You can also check your local suppliers for organic options.

A note about taking care of your skin during treatment: Radiation and chemotherapy pose extra challenges, including reducing natural oils and leaving skin sore, irritated, and very dry. Try to find products that

are designed specifically to sooth and heal treatment-sensitive skin and that are fragrance-free, non-toxic, and alcohol-free. And before you begin using products, be sure to have them checked by your care team: Some lotions may interfere with radiation, and your oncologist may prefer to provide you with or recommend specific products instead.

....

"Awareness is empowering."

—*Rita Wilson, actress, singer, activist,
producer, breast cancer survivor*

SKIN PROBLEMS

Acne

Many types of cancer treatment may cause acne. If you do get acne, you're most likely to get it on your face and head, but it can also appear on other areas of your body. Talk with your doctor before using any over-the-counter products, as they may want you to avoid using them during treatment.

To help treat acne, keep your skin clean. See Chapters 3 and 4 for tips and recommendations.

Recommended Products:

- Apple Cider Vinegar: It's packed with potassium, magnesium, acetic acid, and various enzymes that kill bacteria on the skin. Apply with a cotton ball.
- Oral or topical antibiotics or topical steroids as they can reduce inflammation and speed healing.

Blistering Skin

Consult your medical team.

Dry/Cracked Skin

Recommended Products:
- Aveeno Skin Relief Body Wash
- Dove Sensitive Skin Beauty Bar
- Ivory Liquid Body Soap
- Lindi Skin Body Lotion
- Neutrogena Facial Moisturizer
- 100% Virgin Coconut Oil
- Aquaphor Healing Ointment
- Aveeno Intense Relief Hand Cream
- CeraVe Moisturizing Cream
- Ocean Bottom Soap Company (organic soaps and moisturizers)

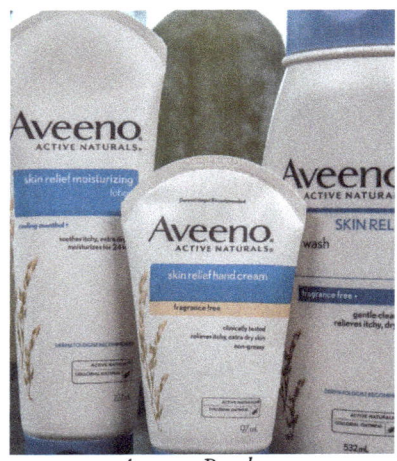

Aveeno Products

Flushing/Red Cheeks

This is usually caused by steroids and will typically go away on its own. If you use a foundation or powder with green undertones, this will usually neutralize the red tones.

Recommended Products:

- Clinique Redness Solutions Make-up
- Clinique Redness Solutions Pressed Powder

Photosensitivity

Photosensitivity, or the tendency to sunburn easily, can happen with some cancer therapies.

Avoid the sun for any length of time; but if you need to be outdoors, there are many ways to protect your skin. The Skin Cancer Foundation recommends protective clothing, a wide-brimmed UPF hat, gloves, UV-blocking sunglasses, and being in the shade whenever possible.

It is also a good idea to ask your doctor to recommend a sunscreen for sensitive skin if your skin is irritated anywhere from radiation therapy. This area will be the most sensitive to sunburn, especially during the first year after treatment.

Keep any surgical scars covered from the sun, as surgical scars may be especially sensitive to sun damage. If you can't keep them covered by clothes (or a hat), apply sunscreen with a broad-spectrum SPF of 30 or higher, generously and frequently.

Recommended Products:

- Coolibar Protective Clothing
- Garnier Ombrelle Complete Lotion SPF 30
- Neutrogena Sheer Zinc Dry Touch Sunscreen Broad Spectrum SPF 50

Puffy Eyes

Puffy eyes can be treated naturally with cold cucumber slices, tea bags, or aloe vera. And here are a few other product-based solutions my clients have used.

Recommended Products:

- Vichy Aqualia Thermal Eye Roll-On
- Garnier Anti-Puff Eye Roller

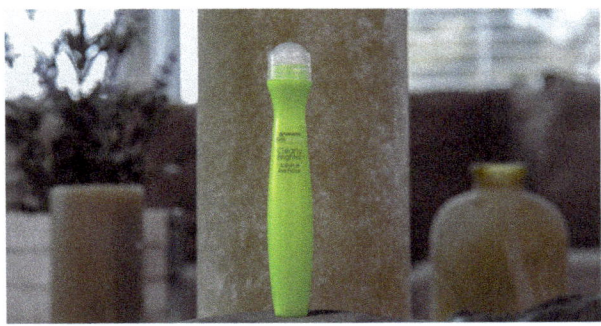

Garnier Anti-Puff Eye Roller

Radiation Burns

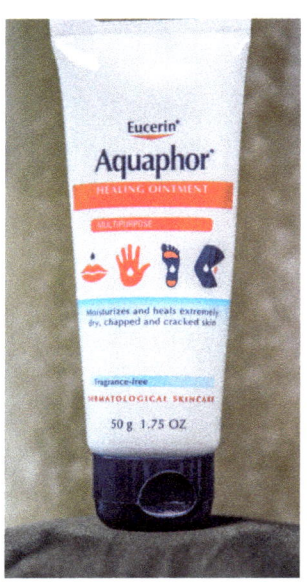

*Aquaphor
Healing Ointment*

Contact your medical team immediately if you see signs of burning. Radiation burn—also called radiation recall—may take weeks to appear, if it appears at all. It's a sunburn-like rash. More severe symptoms may include redness, tenderness, swelling, wet sores, and peeling skin. Contact your care team immediately if any of these symptoms occur. They may prescribe a corticosteroid. I was told as well that there are studies that have shown a mild prescription-strength topical steroid applied daily starting the first day of radiation can decrease the severity of symptoms.

Try to avoid further irritation. Wear loose-fitting clothes. Avoid harsh products: Find some designed to specifically sooth and heal treatment-sensitive skin and that are fragrance free, non-toxic, and alcohol free.

If you are experiencing only a slight irritation, these products have helped my clients:

- Aquaphor Healing Ointment
- Jeans Cream—a vitamin and plant extract blend
- Lindi Skin—Cooler Roll, Cooler Pad, Soothing Balm, Body Wash
- Ocean Bottom Soap Company—Lotion Bars

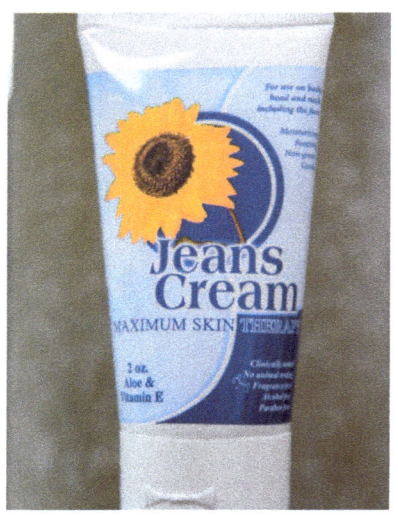

Jeans Cream

Rashes/Hives/Itching

Be sure to report these to your medical team at onset. In many cases, they can be resolved or minimized. It may be as simple as using a cold compress, aloe vera, and hydrating moisturizer. If this is not effective, a prescription drug may be necessary.

Recommended Products:
- Aveeno Skin Relief Soothing Body Wash
- Aveeno Skin Relief Soothing Bath Treatment
- Lindi Body Lotion

Skin Discoloration

Skin discoloration will usually resolve itself post-treatment. If not, you may want to see a dermatologist once you have completed all treatment and are on the mend. They may suggest laser treatment or skin bleaching.

SCARRING

"Never be ashamed of a scar. It simply means that you were stronger than whatever tried to hurt you."
—Unknown

Scars are a natural part of the body's healing process. All surgeries will leave some scarring, and the level of severity varies widely from person to person. For example, your age, race, genetics, and the size of your incision can make a difference in how well you heal. Some things are beyond anyone's control while other factors could help make the

scars less visible. Most will fade naturally over time but will never go away completely.

Discuss any concerns about scarring with your surgeon. In some situations, you may be able to choose in which direction you prefer the incision to be made. For example, you may be a candidate for a horizontal incision with abdomen surgery; in most cases, a horizontal scar of this kind can be concealed under panties or swimwear.

Types of Scars

Keloid

Keloid scars develop when scar tissue forms in excessive amounts and occur as a result of surgery. This type of scarring is found predominantly in people with dark skin, but anyone could develop it. Generally, they aren't harmful, but they can produce discomfort. They can be pink to red in color and can be itchy, tender, and painful. The visual appearance of a keloid scar is smooth. It looks almost like a second skin is developing on or around the scar site.

Hypertrophic

Hypertrophic scars and keloid scars occur for the same reason: The body is over-producing collagen to compensate for the wound. But hypertrophic and keloid scars differ in appearance significantly. Hypertrophic scarring will become raised and remain at the incision site, whereas keloid scars can become quite enlarged and can appear both at the site and around it. Hypertrophic scars are what you will have after a lumpectomy, mastectomy and/or reconstruction, and they tend to fade over time.

Contractured

This type of scar mostly occurs after radiation therapy. The scar tightens the skin, which can impair your mobility and may affect muscles and nerves.

There are medical and non-medical ways to treat scarring. I suggest you consult with a dermatologist or cosmetic surgeon to discuss your options before beginning any treatment.

Reducing the Appearance of Scars

Always practice proper wound care by following the instructions of your surgeon. If you see any sign of infection, contact your surgeon immediately. An infection could contribute to more serious scarring.

In addition, doing the following can help your skin heal more effectively and help reduce scarring:

- Refrain from smoking
- Avoid alcohol
- Drink plenty of water
- Eat well
- Avoid sun exposure

Over-the-Counter Scar Treatments

Dermaflage

> Scar and Wrinkle Filler: Their scar removal kit includes an applicator, texture pad, mixing tools, mixing tips, and instructions for a 30-day supply of concealer in your selected tone.

> Scar Removal Cream: Their Good Skin product is quickly absorbed into the skin and suitable for all skin types. It improves the appearance of scars and works as a moisturizer and make-up primer.

Mederma

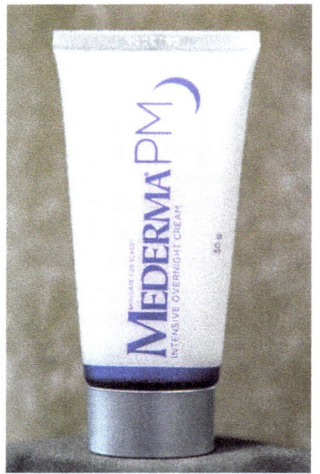

Mederma PM

Mederma PM: This is an intensive overnight cream.

Quick Dry Oil: This oil combines cepalin with botanicals in a paraben-free and dye-free formulation.

Advanced Scar Gel: This is a once-a-day formulated scar care product clinically shown to reduce the appearance of scars, both old and new.

Scar Away

Silicone Scar Sheets: These work to flatten, soften, and fade new and old scars while minimizing the formation of new scars. It also conceals while you heal.

Silicone Scar Gel: This 100 percent silicone scar gel is formulated using patented, transparent, self-drying silicone gel technology.

Ocean Bottom Soap Company Lotion Bars

Many women have used these with remarkable results. Choose from lavender or unscented lotion bars, as well as bars with essential oils, like frankincense or balsam copaiba, which also help with pain.

Tattoo Art

You can turn surgery scars into a work of art, like Soul Sister Trish did here:

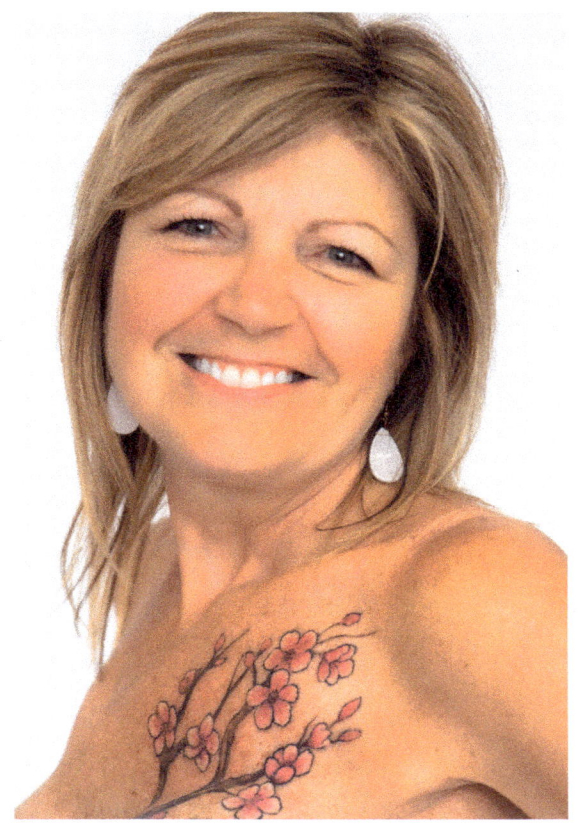

Trish proudly shows off her beautiful tattoo

Please also see Chapter 8 to learn about nipple and areola tattooing.

Alternative Therapy

Massage

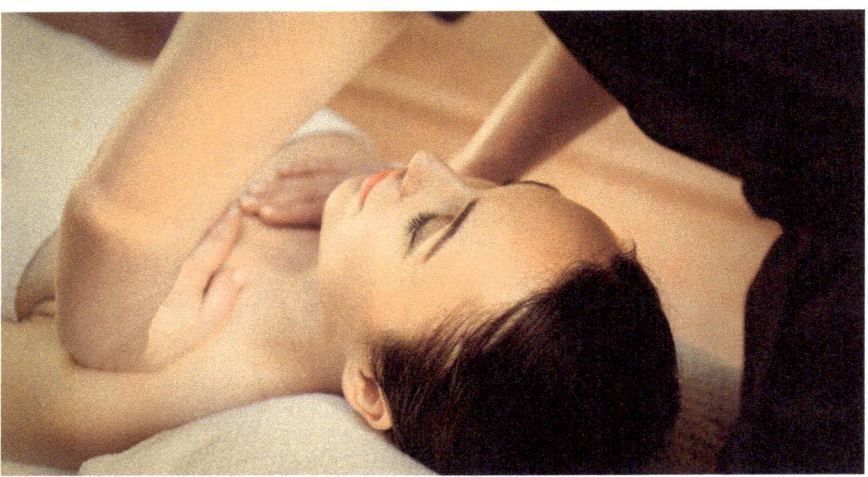

Since the implications of scarring aren't only cosmetic—pain and tightness can also result—professionals are sometimes needed to help ease the patient's scar tissue into a healthier healing pattern. By using vigorous, deep, and soft-tissue massage, massage therapists may help to relieve the pain and feelings of constriction. Please check with your medical team before proceeding with this type of massage.

Yoga

Yoga is deep breathing and whole-body stretches. It can help break up scar tissue and aid in mobility.

Acupuncture

Acupuncture can help reduce tension in the muscles surrounding scar tissue to help reduce pain, encourage healing, and help flatten the appearance of a scar.

Vitamin E Cream

Fresh Aloe

Medical Solutions

You may be a candidate for one or more of the following procedures to help minimize the appearance of your scarring. Please consult a licensed professional to see which might work best for you.

Steroid Injections: These may help to flatten the appearance of the scar.

Collagen Injections: These help to raise sunken scars to the level of healthy, undamaged skin.

Dermabrasion: This involves the removal of the surface layer of skin.

Fractional Resurfacing Laser: Beams are used to break down sections of the scar tissue, causing the skin to regenerate with healthy, undamaged skin.

Botox: Treating a facial wound in the early healing phase with botulinum toxin could improve the appearance of a scar later on.

MOUTH PROBLEMS

Dry Mouth

Chemotherapy and radiation therapy can cause dry mouth by damaging the salivary glands. Not only does saliva act like a lubricant, it also contains enzymes that break down bacteria that cause cavities. It acts like an infection fighter, which is especially critical when going through treatment. This is why it's so important to keep your mouth lubricated.

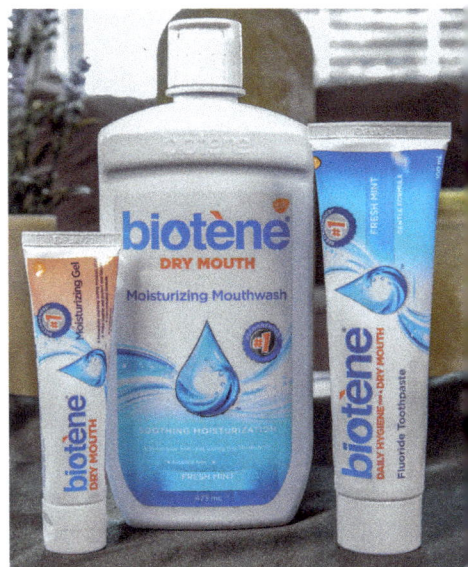

Biotène Products

Recommended Products:

- Biotène—Moisturizing Gel, Mouthwash, Toothpaste
- PerioSciences AO ProRinse Hydrating Mouthwash, Hydrating Dry Mouth AO Pro Gel
- Salagen—a prescription drug
- SalivaSure—saliva substitute lozenges

Oral Thrush

Most people have oral thrush, which is caused by the fungus candida, a normal organism in your mouth. Oral candidiasis usually doesn't cause any problems, but when your immune system is weakened, there's a greater chance of developing an overgrowth of the fungus. A white coating (lesion) on your tongue is a good indication. Probiotics can help with oral thrush, but ask your medical team if this is something you can take. They may choose to prescribe an antifungal medication instead, or nothing at all.

Metallic Taste

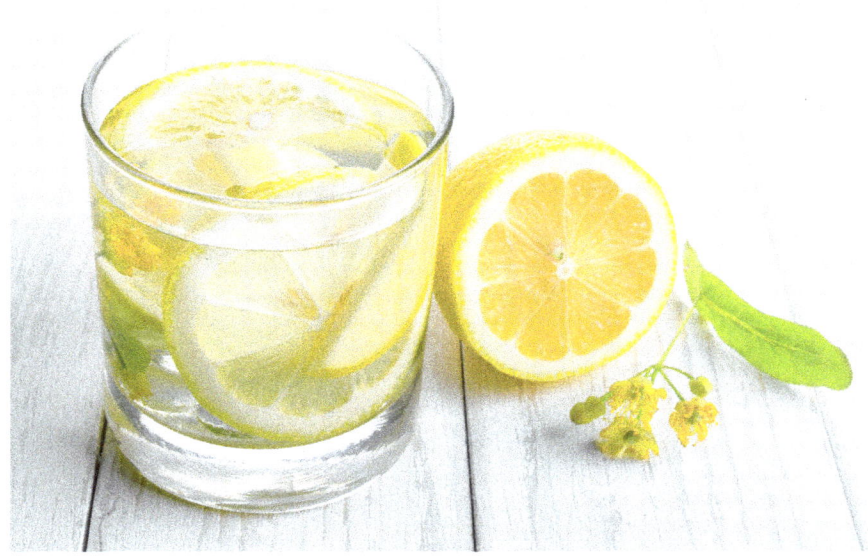

A metallic taste, or other taste change, is quite common during cancer treatment. Add fresh lemon to water for flavor or a splash of 100 percent juice. You can try rinsing your mouth with ginger ale, tea, or salted water before eating to clear your taste buds. Also, try using plastic utensils rather than metal. Many of my clients find lemon candies also do the trick.

Mouth Sores

Rinse your mouth with plain water or soda water or add a touch of salt or baking soda. Lip balm will help with dry, cracked lips. Eat chilled or frozen foods, like milkshakes, ice creams, and popsicles. Sucking on small frozen fruit such as grapes is also a great way to soothe your mouth and get nutrients at the same time. Avoid mouthwashes that contain alcohol or hydrogen peroxide as both are too harsh while in treatment. Sucking on ice cubes right before infusions may help prevent mouth sores.

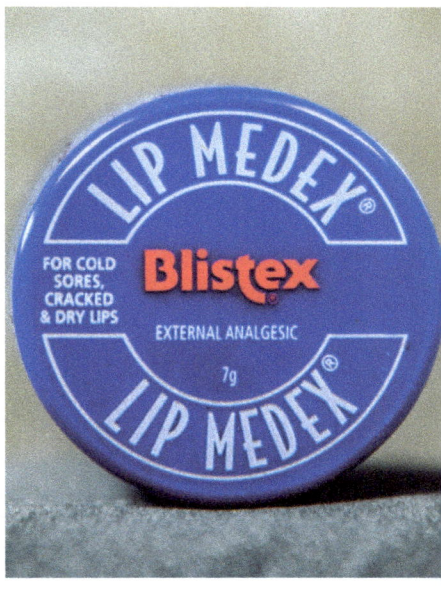

Blistex Lip Medex

Recommended Products:

- Biotène—Toothpaste, Moisturizing Mouthwash
- Blistex Lip MedEx

OTHER SIDE EFFECTS

Gas and Bloating

Surgeries such as hysterectomies and certain chemotherapies can potentially lead to embarrassing gas and bloating. This can be uncomfortable and cause belching and flatulence. Needless to say, this could make you feel less ladylike. Here are some suggestions that can help

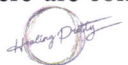

stimulate gut motility. Your medical team can tell you if these recommendations could be beneficial for you and your individual needs.

- Use a warm pack on your belly. However, if you have an incision in this area, be sure to stay away from direct skin contact and, of course, make sure it's not too hot.
- Walk
- Sip on warm drinks
- Avoid gas-producing foods
- Take probiotics (check with your doctor first)
- Try Gas-X tablets (check with your doctor first)

Nausea

Some chemotherapy drugs are more likely to cause nausea and vomiting than others. Take any anti-nausea medicines as your doctor recommends. If your doctor hasn't prescribed medicines for you, you could ask about taking a non-prescription anti-nausea medicine, such as:

- Dimenhydrinate (Gravol)
- An antihistamine, such as Benadryl

Another alternative is Nabilone. This is a pill that has synthetic cannabinoids. Cannabinoids are chemicals that act on certain receptors on cells in the body, especially cells in the central nervous system. It's sometimes given to people with cancer if standard anti-nausea drugs do not help relieve these symptoms.

Here are some other ways to help when you have a queasy feeling. Some of these suggestions have been taken from the Canadian Cancer Society website:

"I laughed more in the hospital than I ever have in my life, making fun of all the weird things that were happening to me. My friends

would walk in with this sad look, and I would
throw something at them and say, 'Come on!
This isn't the end of the world!"
—*Christina Applegate, actress, comedian, dancer,*
breast cancer survivor

- Try eating three to four hours before treatment, and *not* right before treatment (if necessary, have a light snack before treatment). Wait a few hours after treatment before eating again. Eat before getting hungry, because hunger can increase nausea.

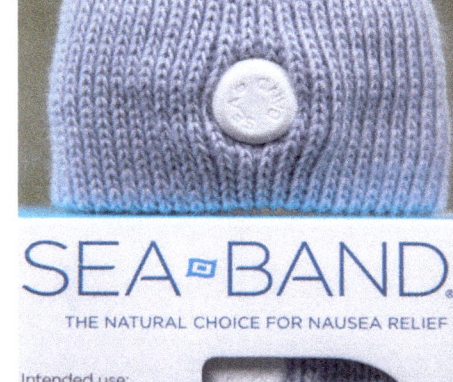

THE NATURAL CHOICE FOR NAUSEA RELIEF

Intended use:
The Sea-Band Ltd
"Sea-Band"
is indicated for
the relief of nausea

Sea-Band Wrist Band

- Avoid mixing hot and cold foods during the same meal. Serve food cold or at room temperature to reduce strong tastes and smells.
- Avoid having liquids with meals. Drink fluids 30 minutes *before* a meal, rather than *with* the meal. Sip water, juices, and other caffeine-free liquids (flat ginger ale, sport drinks, etc.) throughout the day. Cool liquids may be easier to drink than very hot or very cold liquids. Try to drink at least eight to ten glasses of fluid each day to help prevent dehydration if vomiting.
- Avoid foods that are overly sweet, greasy, fried, or spicy, or that have strong smells.
- Eat small meals often throughout the day. Nibble on dry or bland foods, such as crackers, toast, dry cereals, bread sticks, pretzels, bagels, potatoes, or yogurt when waking up and also every few hours during the day.
- Consume clear liquids (such as flat soda, broth, juice, etc.)
- Don't lie down for at least two hours after meals.

- Try ginger gum, ginger ale.

You also may want to try Sea Bands. They are acupressure bands that fit around your wrist. A plastic stud is attached to the inside of the wristband, which exerts pressure and stimulates the P6 (or *Nei-Kuan*) acupressure point. The pressure may relieve nausea and vomiting.

Hot Flashes

Hot flashes and night sweats may be a result of the type of cancer you have, certain cancer drugs, or other conditions.

Here are a few tips that may be helpful.

- Some women have had success with herbs and dietary supplements such as Vitamin E, soy and black cohosh, ground flaxseed, dong quai, milk thistle, red clover, licorice root extract, and chaste tree berry. A note of caution that soy contains estrogen-like substances and the effect of soy on the risk of breast cancer growth or reoccurrence isn't clear at this point. Be sure to tell your medical team if you are taking or planning to take natural supplements.
- Stress and anxiety treatments. Talk to your medical team about what is referred to as psychosocial interventions.
- Hypnosis is a newer treatment for hot flashes, and some women have had good success.
- Dressing in layers is always smart.
- Try to keep your weight within normal range. Extra pounds can make hot flashes more severe.
- Avoid caffeine, spicy foods, and alcohol to help minimize hot flashes.
- Please see Chapter 8 for hot-flash friendly clothing.

Inflammation/Swelling

Fluid retention, called edema, is swelling caused by the abnormal buildup of fluid in the body. Edema is most common in the feet and

legs. It can also occur in the hands, arms, face, and abdomen. Some types of chemotherapy can cause edema. To help reduce swelling and relieve symptoms, eat a well-balanced diet, limit the amount of salt in your diet, walk or do other exercises (ask your health care team to recommend some). Also talk with your health care team about wearing special stockings, sleeves, or gloves that help with circulation if your swelling is severe.

Cognitive Impairment ("Chemo Brain")

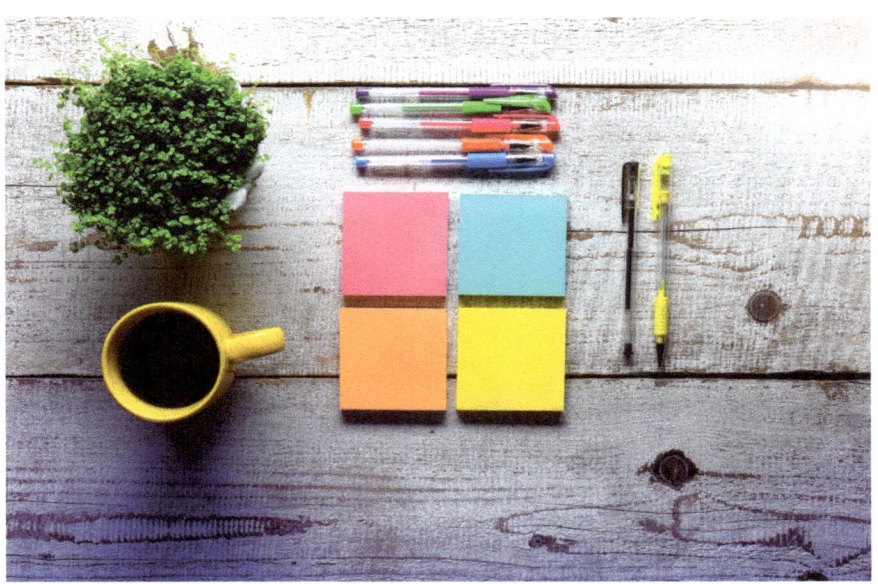

You may develop cognitive impairment, better known as "chemo brain," while undergoing treatment. Understanding that "it's not just you" can bring some comfort if this happens. You may forget things you already know or forget what you were going to do, have trouble concentrating, lose your train of thought, have trouble multi-tasking, or feel "slow" in your thinking and mental processing. Medical researchers have not yet determined when or why this happens, but it's a common side effect. Talk to your medical team about any concerns you may have. And here are some tips to help you get through:

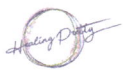

- Use a planner or smart phone to keep track of your appointments
- Keep sticky notes handy—write down what you need to remember.
- Do one thing at a time.
- Repeat aloud, and often, what you'd like to remember.
- Get lots of rest and sleep.
- Exercise. Even a slow walk can help you feel more alert.
- Keep your brain in shape too. Try completing brain games like puzzles or crosswords.
- Eat healthy foods like vegetables and Omega-3-rich foods to help keep up your brain power.
- People always want to help. Don't forget to ask for help.

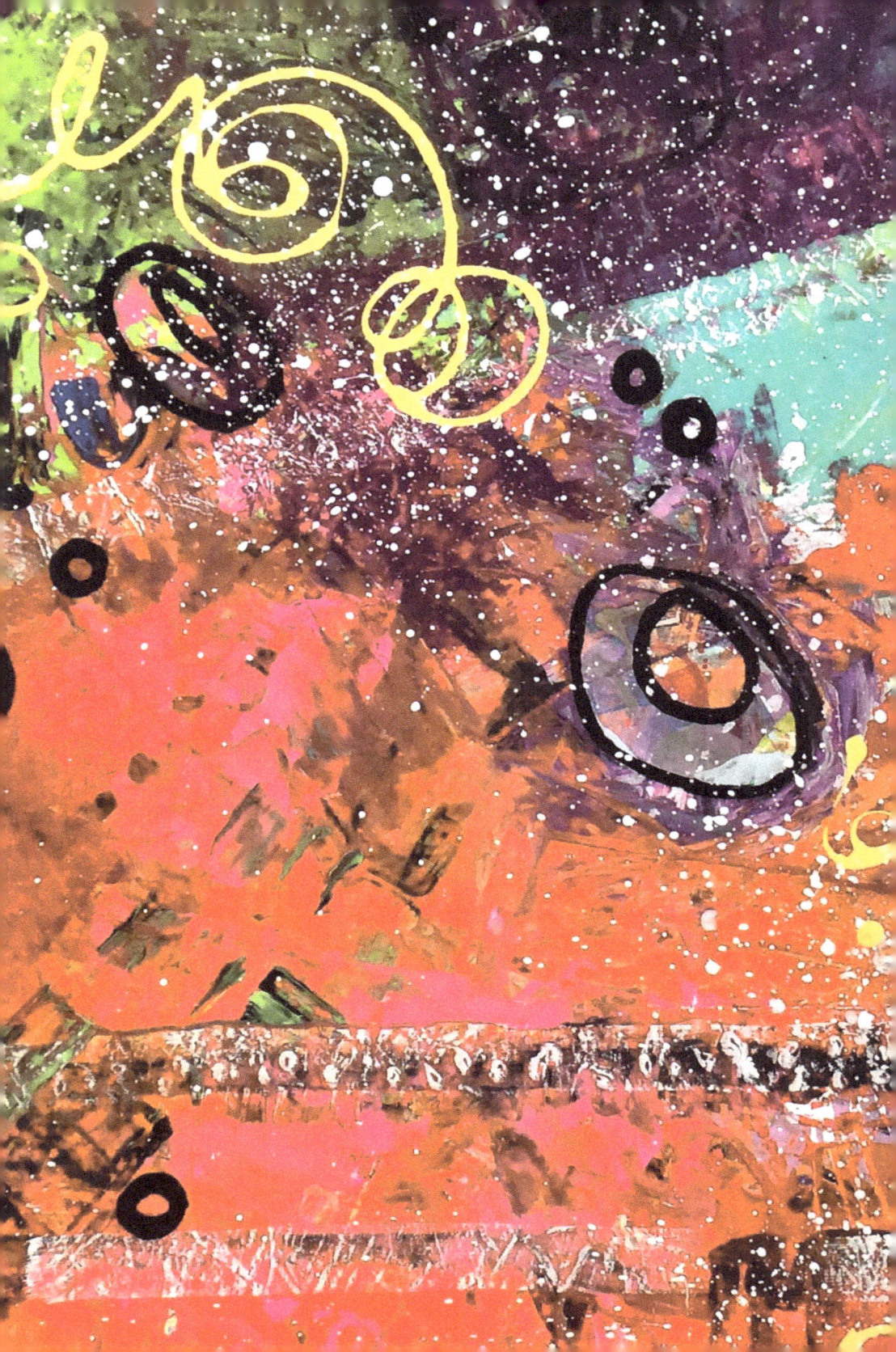

"Now I have a third must-do on my list of things to do with cancer, and it's this: Follow your gut, ask questions, and don't be complacent."

—Cynthia Nixon, actress, activist, politician, breast cancer survivor

. . . .

7

Surgery Smarts

Preparing for surgery

In my experience, knowing what to expect can help you feel more comfortable and reduce your stress about your surgery.

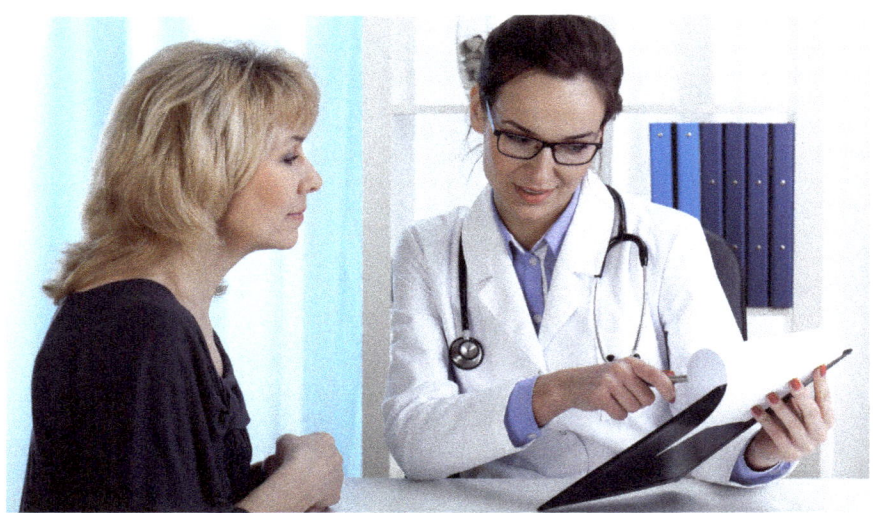

It's very important that you know your options. Your healthcare provider should clearly explain the surgical procedure you're about to undergo. Take notes, and don't hesitate to ask the same questions until you completely understand. Get printed material about your condition and surgery, and

review it thoroughly. Ask if there are different methods for doing this operation and why your surgeon favors one way over another. Don't leave yourself with any doubts, and consider getting a second opinion.

Many women are sent home after surgery not knowing that there were products that could have benefitted them. Ask your surgeon what to expect. Find out if there are special supplies, equipment, or healing aids that will help you once you're home, and make sure these items are purchased beforehand and ready to use. As an example, many of my mastectomy and lumpectomy clients weren't aware of post-surgical healing bras, which are a must-have item after surgery. See Chapter 8 for more information about these bras.

Also, ask how long a full recovery is expected to take, and know what limitations will be placed on you. Knowing these things ahead of time will help you feel more in control.

CHECKLIST

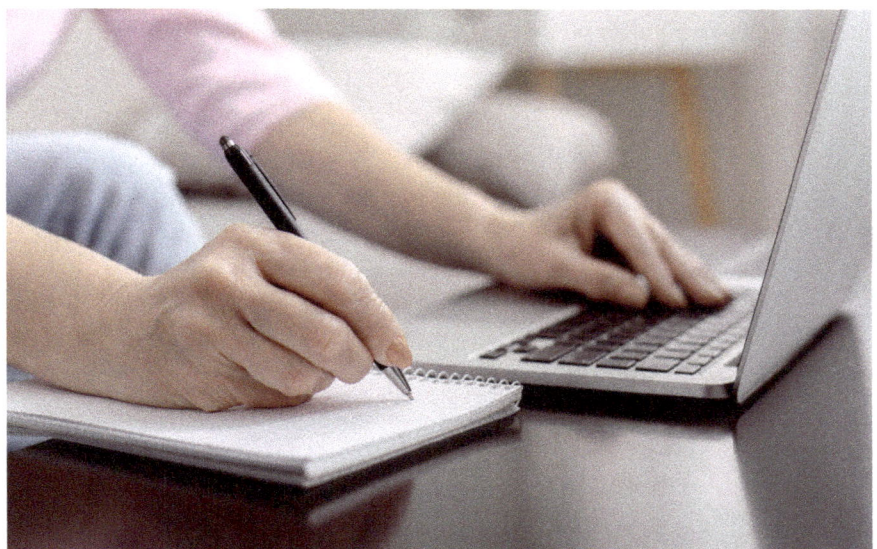

Here's a handy list of hospital essentials to bring with you:

- Picture ID
- Health Insurance ID card
- List of your medications
- Advanced directives/Living will
- Reading glasses (if needed)
- Earplugs
- Sleep mask
- Time-passers, such as a copy of *Healing Pretty*, other books, magazines, e-reader, iPad, etc.
- Cell phone & charger
- Toiletries, including lip balm
- Specialty post-op clothing and products that are comfortable and can accommodate any bandages, drains, or swelling that you may have
- Seat belt pillow
- Favorite robe, slippers, cozy blanket

And finally, if possible, talk to women who have been through similar surgeries. There are many support groups who would love to share their stories and guide you through it.

COMFORTING WORDS FROM AN OPERATING ROOM NURSE

While writing *Healing Pretty*, I consulted with my dear friend Linda Moroun, a registered nurse of 40 years (who has since retired) whose opinion I greatly value. Linda practiced much of her career as an OR nurse. In her own words, here's what Linda feels you should know before going into surgery.

Linda's Story

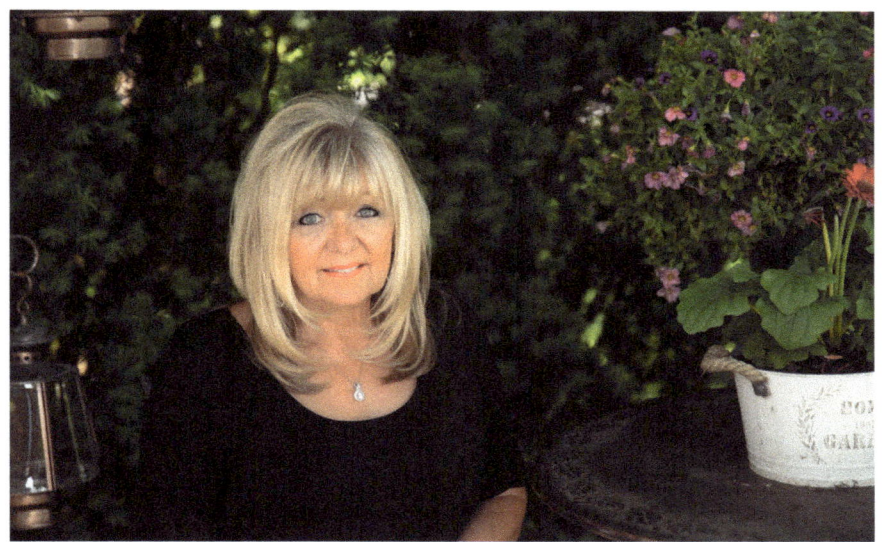

Linda Moroun

Having worked as an OR nurse for 25 years, I'd like to share with you some insight into what we do as medical professionals to make you feel comfortable and confident before and during your surgery.

You'll have a team of doctors and nurses concentrating only on your well being. In my experience, your team will consist of your surgeon, an assisting physician, an anesthesiologist, a scrub nurse, and a circulating nurse.

Your team will ask you many questions repeatedly, as each person wants a clear understanding of you and your history. It helps to have your information written down, such as current medications and supplements, previous surgeries, drug allergies, environmental sensitivities, and any medical and psychological conditions you may have.

A sterile environment is of utmost importance, and respect for tissue is always their imperative.

The care team is very sensitive to the anxieties of patients and their families. We truly do care—we've all had family members that have experienced similar significant events, and even had some ourselves. Remember, nurses and doctors went into the medical profession to help people.

Lastly, I'd like to share with you my favorite work in the operating room: giving my patients a warm blanket before surgery, comforting and reassuring them while holding their hand as they fall asleep.

Thank you for allowing me to share. You will be in good hands.

Linda Moroun, 2019

TYPES OF SURGERIES

Face, Head, and Neck

If cancer is removed from your face, you'll find some helpful information and resources in Chapters 4 and 6.

There are several cancers of the head and neck that may require surgery. If you're having surgery on your head or brain, some of your hair will likely be shaved. Your hair should grow back, but you may have a noticeable bare spot on your head for a while. Please refer to Chapter 2 for hair-loss solutions.

Other cancers such as throat, larynx, and thyroid could result in a visible neck scar. Scarring creams, make-up, and avoiding the sun are beneficial. You can also use fashion to camouflage this type of scar. Please refer to Chapter 8 for helpful tips.

Breast

Lumpectomy

Lumpectomy is the removal of the breast tumor (the "lump") and some of the normal tissue that surrounds it.

Lumpectomy is a form of "breast-conserving" or "breast preservation" surgery. There are several names used for breast-conserving surgery, such as biopsy, lumpectomy, partial mastectomy, re-excision, quadrantectomy, or wedge resection. Technically, a lumpectomy is a partial mastectomy because part of the breast tissue is removed. But the amount of tissue removed can vary greatly; for example, a quadrantectomy means that roughly a quarter of your breast will be removed. Make sure you have a clear understanding from your surgeon about how much of your breast may be gone after surgery, and what kind of scar you will have.

Mastectomy

A mastectomy is the surgical removal of the entire breast. If you have a mastectomy, you may choose to use a prosthetic to replace the breast that was removed, or you may want to have some type of reconstruction to replace the breast.

Breast pillows are very nice and comforting healing aids, as surgical incision sites can sometimes be bothersome. Breast pillows are soft, U-shaped pillows that rest under the pit of your arm, making them great items to use while lounging or sleeping. My clients say this pillow is a must-have.

Reconstruction

Reconstruction, of course, is a very personal choice, and one that should be researched thoroughly. There are many reasons why a woman would opt for reconstruction: Perhaps you feel uncomfortable with your mastectomy scar; or you don't want to live flat or asymmetrical; or you feel that a prosthetic would be uncomfortable; or you want to

return to something near your original physical appearance. You will want to look at whatever will give you increased self-confidence.

....

"(My breasts) are fabulous! Mine aren't even teenagers yet!"

—Sharon Osbourne, television host, entrepreneur, author, breast cancer survivor

Here are some things to keep in mind when you are making your decision.

If you opt for reconstruction, it may be performed immediately following your mastectomy, called "immediate reconstruction," or you may be advised to wait, which is termed "delayed reconstruction."

Immediate reconstruction reduces the need for multiple surgeries; however, if you're having expanders put in, then you will still need an additional surgery to change the expander to an implant. Often the cosmetic results are better; however, it's important to know that it's a longer surgery than doing them as two separate procedures, and it also involves a longer recovery time.

Delayed reconstruction may be medically necessary if additional treatment, such as radiation, is required after a mastectomy. Delayed reconstruction gives you the benefit of more time to research reconstruction options and to make reconstruction decisions at a later date, allowing you to focus exclusively on cancer treatments for the time being. However, cosmetic results may not be as good as immediate reconstruction.

There are three types of breast reconstruction options available: autologous reconstruction, implant-based reconstruction, and hybrid reconstruction.

Autologous Reconstruction: This procedure involves using tissue from other parts of the body to reconstruct the breast. Most of the time, the tissue used comes from the belly, buttocks, inner thighs, or back.

Implant-based Reconstruction: This uses a silicone shell filled with saline (salt water), silicone gel, or a combination of the two to rebuild the breast. If you're having implant reconstruction immediately after your mastectomy, and there is enough skin tissue left after the surgery, the implant can be directly inserted below the chest muscle at that time.

Hybrid Reconstruction: This combines the techniques of using other body tissues with a small breast implant. This is usually done when there isn't enough tissue that can be taken from another part of the body to get the desired shape and size for the new breast.

If you will be having a mastectomy or reconstructive surgery, surgical healing kits and compression bras will help you recover with comfort and dignity. Please see Chapter 8 for more information.

Lymph Node Removal

A number of my clients were not aware of lymphedema until they were diagnosed with it. Women and their doctors are focused on taking care of the cancer (rightfully so), and in my experience, lymphedema doesn't seem to get discussed in very much detail at times.

When lymph nodes under your arm (called axillary lymph nodes) are removed during breast surgery or are treated with radiation, some of the lymph vessels can become blocked. This may prevent lymph fluid from leaving the area. Lymphedema occurs when lymph fluid collects in the arm (or other area such as the hand, fingers, chest/breast or back), causing it to swell (edema). Lymphedema can appear in some people months, or even years, after treatment ends.

The best time to take steps to reduce your risk of lymphedema is before breast cancer surgery. Here are the steps, many of them recommended by BreastCancer.org:

- Ask if you might be a candidate for a sentinel lymph node biopsy (SLNB). This is a less invasive procedure that typically removes two to four of the lymph nodes. The more complete axillary lymph node dissection (ALND) takes out many more. Also, if they find cancer cells in the first one or two nodes, ask your surgeon what he or she recommends as a next step. Research has shown that for some women with early-stage breast cancer, axillary lymph node dissection may not be necessary if there are only small amounts of cancer. Radiation therapy, chemotherapy, hormonal therapy, and/or other treatments may be enough to kill the remaining cancer cells. However, if the breast cancer has spread into multiple nodes, your surgeon will likely have to take them out regardless because it reduces the risk of recurrence or spread of the cancer.
- There is a new procedure called axillary reverse mapping (ARM). It uses special dye to locate the lymph nodes and vessels that drain lymph from the arm and hand. The surgeon then tries to preserve those nodes and vessels as much as possible.
- Have the circumference of (distance around) both your arms measured before surgery. Although lymphedema can affect the breast, chest, and underarm areas, it's more common in the arm or hand on the same side as the breast cancer. Early swelling in the arm can be hard to notice. Ask your doctor or nurse if they can take measurements around your hands and at points along your arms (every few inches from the wrist to elbow to upper arm), followed by regular measurements at the same points after treatment. Or, you can take measurements at home. By having these measurements, you'll be able to notice changes in your arm and hand over time. And measuring both sides is important so you can tell the difference between weight gain, which would increase the size of both arms, and lymphedema, which would affect only one.

- Make an appointment with a medical professional who has been trained in lymphedema management. They can help with a number of things, including taking measurements before your surgery and recommending post-surgery exercises and educating you about the symptoms of lymphedema.

Nipple and Areola Reconstruction

The decision to reconstruct or not to reconstruct the nipple does not have to be made upfront; it may be completed years down the road. At a very minimum, the initial mastectomy surgery must be fully healed before a surgeon will consider nipple reconstruction surgery.

The decision to have this portion completed as a final step in the overall recovery process is also a personal preference.

In some cases, you can have a nipple sparing mastectomy. This is when your own nipple and areola are preserved. This is not as common; however, you may be a candidate. Type of breast cancer, shape, and size play a key role in having this procedure.

The surgeon may take tissue from another part of your body to rebuild the nipple, or the nipple may be recreated by "pinching" or "twisting up" any excess skin on the chest in the area where the new nipple will be formed on the nipple mound. A tiny incision is made, and the surgeon reconstructs the illusion of a nipple from your own tissue (usually from the surrounding tissue). This surgery usually involves a short healing and recovery time.

Hysterectomy

If you have uterine/endometrial, cervical, vaginal, or ovarian cancer, there's a chance you may need a full or partial hysterectomy. These may be done with a surgical incision through the abdomen, or it may be done vaginally. Laparoscopic surgery may be an option. There are many factors involved, and only your medical team will know what is best for you.

"I haven't talked much about being an ovarian cancer survivor because I don't really want to define myself that way."

—*Kathy Bates, actress, director, ovarian cancer survivor*

Ostomy

Rectal, bowel, colon, and some gynecological cancers may result in a surgical ostomy, an artificial opening in your abdomen, which will require you to wear an ostomy bag (a prosthetic device to collect waste or urine). The ostomy bag is often temporary, but in some cases, it can be permanent.

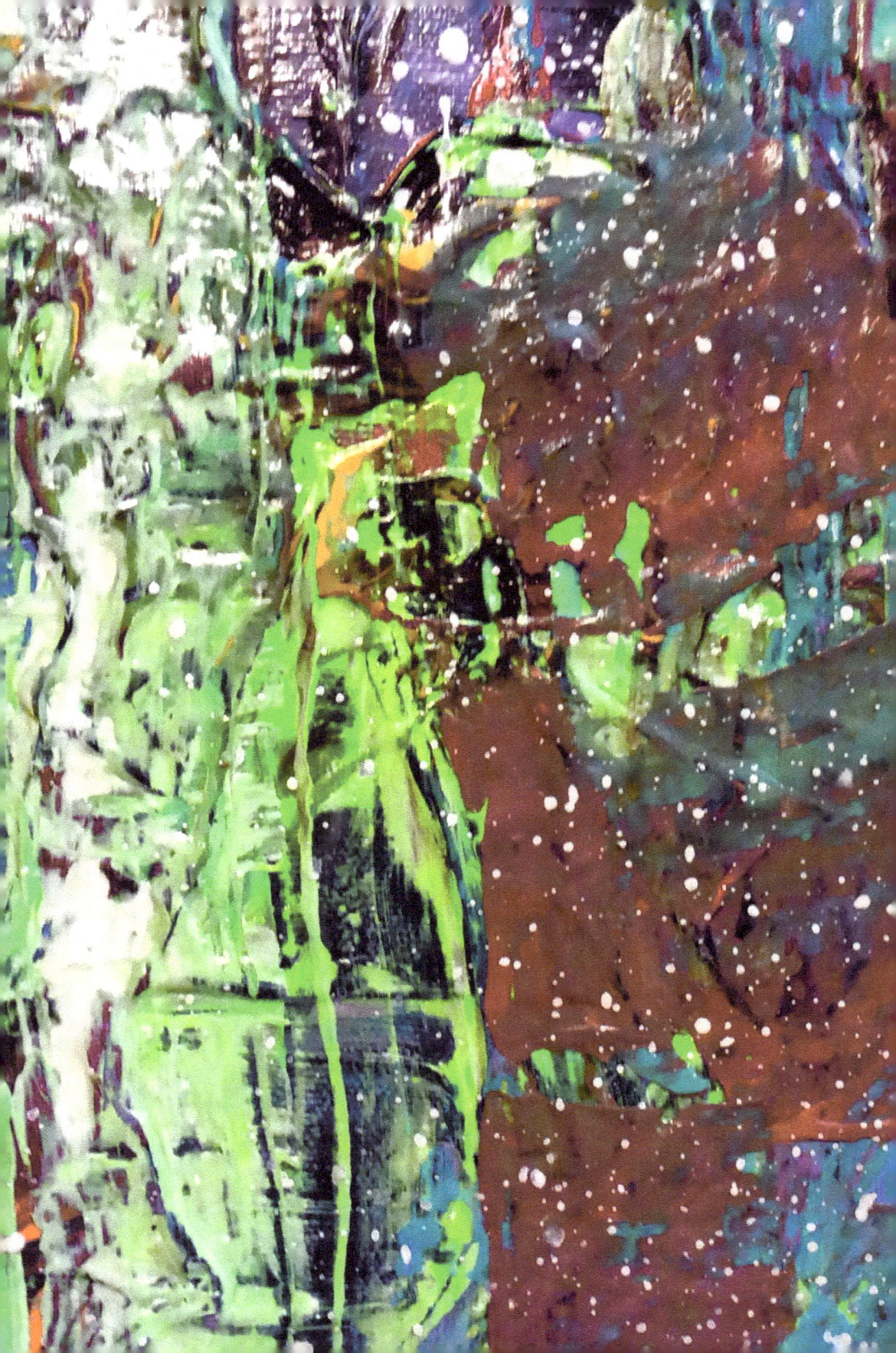

"My whole life has been about changing negatives into positives. I got famous, then I got cancer, and now I live to talk about it. Sometimes the best gifts come in the ugliest packages."

—Fran Drescher, film and television comedian, model, actress, producer, author, activist, uterine cancer survivor

. . . .

8
Practical, Comfy, Pretty, and Funky

Treatment-friendly fashion, accessories, and ideas

Here we cover everything you need to dress with style and to bring you comfort, functionality, and grace during treatment and recovery.

MASTECTOMY, LUMPECTOMY, AND RECONSTRUCTION SOLUTIONS

Bras

Post-Surgical Healing Bra

These are designed to be worn immediately following surgery for comfort and healing. They come as a kit that includes pouches and soft breast forms.

After having a mastectomy, you'll likely be sent home with one or two drainage tubes, depending on whether you had a single or bilateral mastectomy. These tubes can be awkward and uncomfortable, and your skin will be very sensitive.

The pouches can be placed anywhere on the bra to accommodate the drainage tubes. The soft, lightweight breast form can be used until you get a fitting for a prosthetic or until you begin reconstruction. Generally, it takes 6–8 weeks before you are able to have a fitting because the skin is very sensitive.

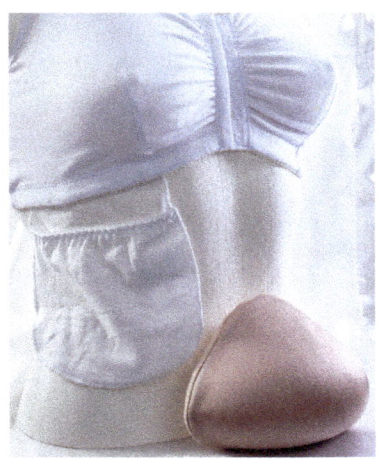

Post-Surgical Healing Kit by American Breast Care

Many women who aren't aware of post-surgical bras remain braless and breastless during this time. In many cases, my clients have told me that they'd wrapped their drainage tubes around their bodies and taped them to their skin, or that they'd tucked them into their pants. Others had stuffed their bra with tissue, not knowing that temporary breast forms were available.

Ask your surgeon if he/she can provide you with these kits, or if he/she could otherwise direct you to where you can find one. My favorite is made by American Breast Care.

Compression

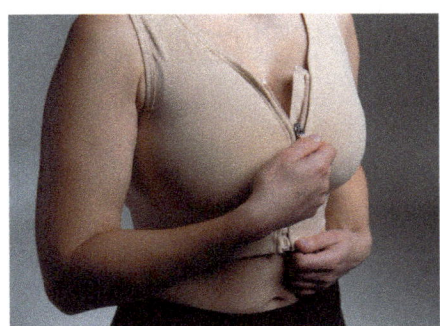

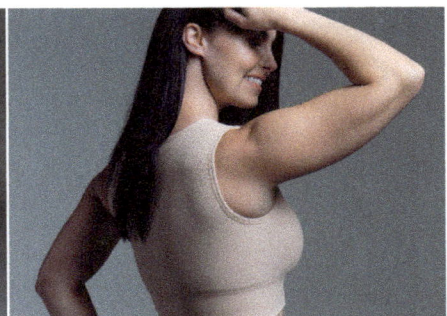

Prairie Hugger compression bra by Prairie Wear (front view)

Prairie Hugger compression bra by Prairie Wear (side/back view)

Compression bras may be necessary to decrease swelling after surgery and to hold the skin in place. Consult with your surgeon before wearing one, as every case is different. My favorite is made by Prairie Wear.

Camisole

A camisole bra is another option for post-surgical recovery, for more comfort and a place for drainage tubes.

Everyday/Mastectomy Bra

In most cases, a mastectomy bra looks just like a regular one. The main difference is the sewn-in pouches designed to hold one or two breast prostheses. With a proper fit, the prosthesis will remain in place while providing you with a sense of security throughout the day and evening.

The bras are also designed to cover scars. Some have a sewn-in camisole to accommodate scars that are higher up or more extensive. Underwire styles do exist but may not be for everyone, depending on the level of sensitivity. A certified mastectomy fitter will be able to assist you.

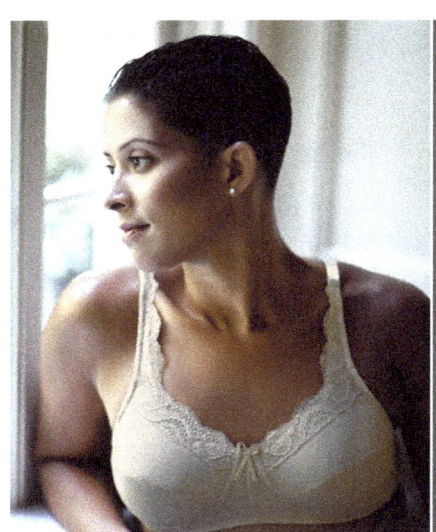 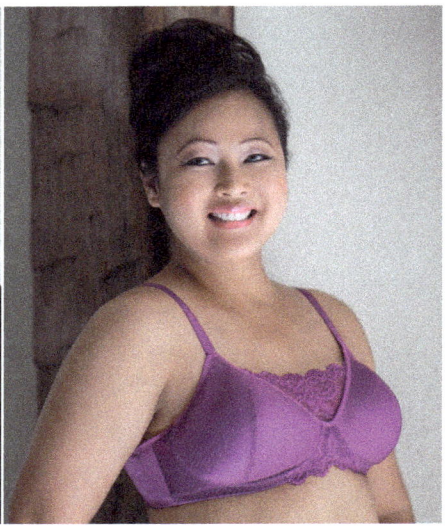

Everyday mastectomy bra by
American Breast Care

Everyday mastectomy camisole bra by
American Breast Care

Prosthetic Options

If you opt not to have reconstructive surgery, there are many prosthetic (artificial) options available. As soon as your healing process is complete, you're ready to be fitted. Some prostheses adhere directly to your skin. They would be a great option for an event to which you plan to wear a backless or strapless dress. Make sure the dress has enough support to hold the prosthesis in place, just in case.

Mastectomy: Full Breast Prosthesis

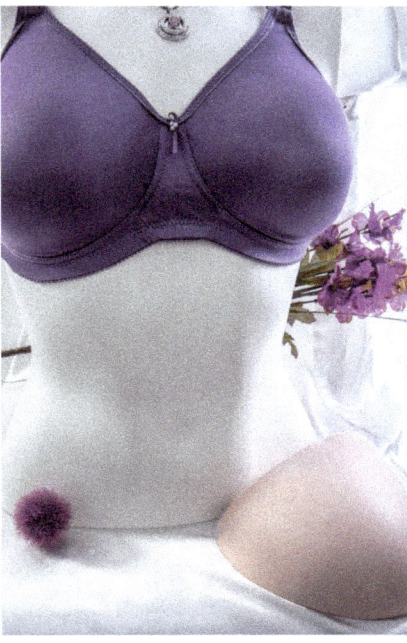

The look, feel, and weight of a breast prosthetic are very similar to a real breast. It's important that your prosthetic is equal to the weight of your natural breast to maintain optimal balance and proportion. Without this, you may develop problems in your neck, shoulders, and back. Just like breasts, prostheses come in all different shapes and sizes, from perky to mature. Make sure you are properly fitted. As much as we would all like the bust of a 20-year-old, it's probably best to stick with something close to what you had pre-surgery, but it all boils down to personal preference.

If you have had a bilateral mastectomy (both breasts), you'll be able to pick any size or shape that you prefer, as long as they are in proportion to your overall body structure. I've observed that larger-breasted women tend to opt for smaller breasts, and smaller-breasted women (you guessed it) opt for larger ones.

Full breast prosthesis (lower right) by American Breast Care

As the old saying goes, we always seem to want what we can't have— except, in this case, we can!

Lumpectomy: Partial Breast Prosthesis

If you have had a lumpectomy, you might be fortunate to not have any visible scarring or indentations. An indentation is how much tissue is taken out at surgery. If your breasts are not proportioned, it can affect your self-esteem. But ladies, there are ways around this too.

"I'm not back to my old self ... and then I realize, I may never get back to my old self. Maybe there's just your new self, your new reality, your new normal. And you make that new normal as good as it can be."

—Joan Lunden, news anchor, author, breast cancer survivor

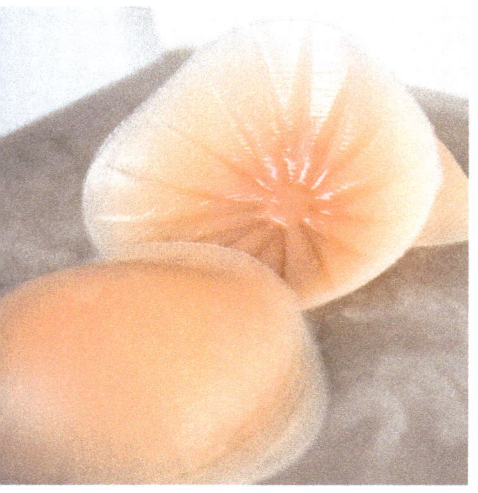

Shapers by American Breast Care

You may want to consider a partial prosthetic to fill in the gap of the lumpectomy site. On the other hand, in some cases, you may need a partial prosthetic to lift or fill in your natural breast. This could occur if you've had reconstruction on only one breast, because as we age, our natural breast could come to sag while the reconstructed breast will remain the same.

Depending upon how much tissue is taken, you may benefit from the comfort of a post-surgical bra (as mentioned earlier).

Shapers are also an option. These are not as full as partial prostheses and are used mostly to restore the appearance of symmetry and balance, as to provide irregular breasts with an even silhouette.

Prosthetics come in a variety of shapes, sizes, colors, and materials, including silicone, micro beads, lightweight foam, or cotton-filled. American Breast Care is my favorite brand.

Swimwear Prosthetics

If you spend a lot of time in the water, I recommend using swim forms, which are used in place of prosthetics. They are specially designed to hold up in water. They also dry faster.

Adhesive Nipples

Sheila Smith, one of my former clients and now a dear friend, shared with me a story that serves as a much-needed reminder of the importance of maintaining a sense of humor.

Sheila's Story

Having gone to sleep with my stick-on nipples, I awoke to find that one of them had disappeared. My husband and I looked for it—under the covers, on the floor, inside my nighty—everywhere! Eventually, we figured it would turn up on its own. But as I turned to walk away from my husband, my husband suddenly burst out laughing—the missing nipple was stuck to my back!

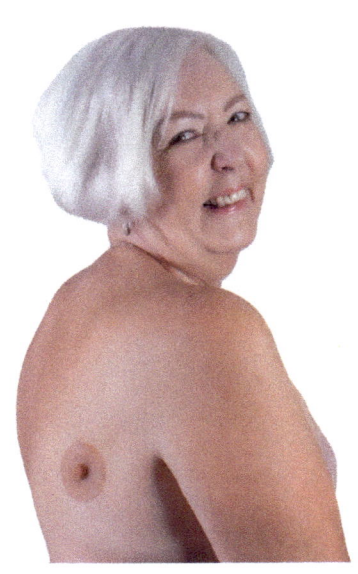

Adhesive nipples are a quick and easy way to create the appearance of realistic nipples and can be worn on reconstructed breasts or directly on your prosthetic. They're a good option—but with prolonged use, they begin to lose their adhesiveness.

Pink Perfect produces realistic custom-made and ready-made adhesive silicone nipples. Their nipple prostheses were designed by an artist and breast cancer survivor. The Pink Perfect adhesive nipple prosthesis replicates the shape, size, color, and texture of your remaining nipple. It is waterproof and can be worn in the shower, ocean, or swimming pool.

Swimwear

Mastectomy swimwear has sewn-in pouches to hold prosthetics. Your local cancer care boutique may carry mastectomy swimwear. If you prefer to shop online, HAPARI has a great selection of mastectomy-friendly swimwear at a reasonable cost.

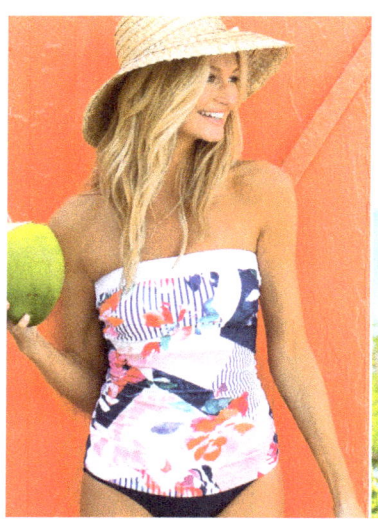

Mastectomy Swimwear
by HAPARI

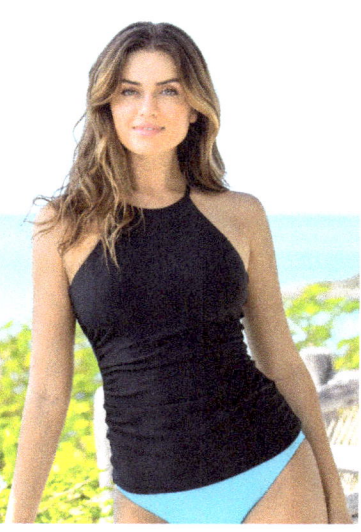

Mastectomy Swimwear
by HAPARI

OSTOMY OPTIONS

Urinary Bag Covers

The ostomy bag is often temporary, but in some cases, it can be permanent. There is a wide selection of fashionable underwear, support belts, urinary bag covers, and ostomy pouches, all in decorative colors and patterns. You can also find stylish swimwear and pretty plugs.

A great product I've discovered is Grandma's Hands. They make ostomy bag covers for one and two-piece bag systems in three fabric choices—cotton, stretchy, and satin—and all are machine washable.

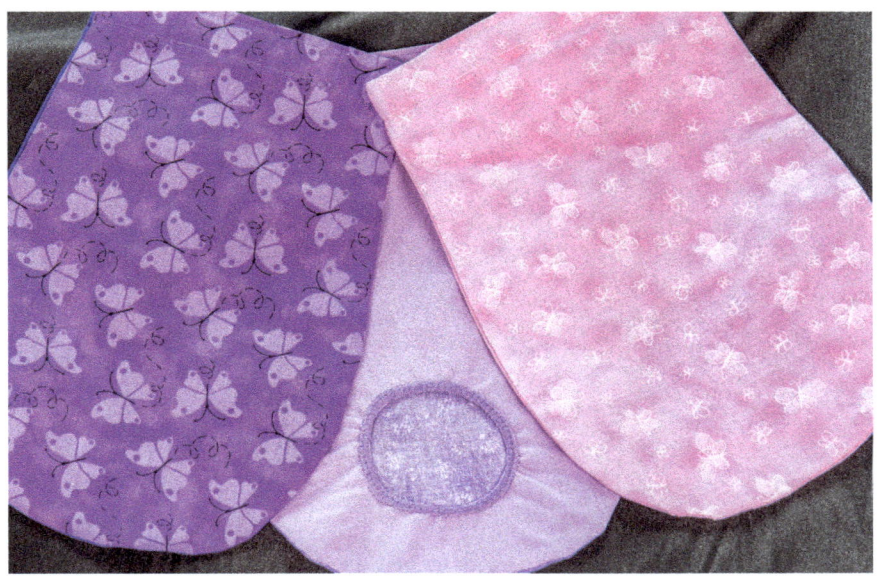

*Ostomy Covers
by Grandma's Hands*

Odor Eliminators

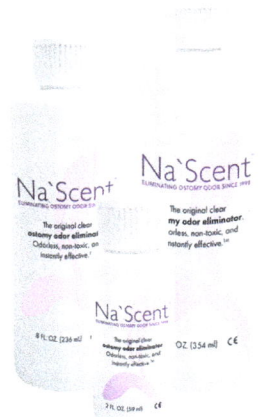

Na 'Scent offers an odor eliminator which kills anaerobic bacteria and enhances hygiene. These products will provide you with comfort and dignity, and they allow you to live an active life with confidence.

And a great online resource is www.veganostomy.ca, which provides ostomy tips, care, product reviews, and more.

Odor Eliminator Products
by Na 'Scent

HYSTERECTOMY RESOURCES

There are many products and resources available to help you feel comfortable and confident after a hysterectomy.

Panties

Specially designed panties can help you feel better sooner after a hysterectomy or other lower abdominal surgery. A great product is the Post Op Panty, which features anatomic medical grade compression to reduce pain, bloating, swelling, and tenderness. It also lets you get back to your normal activities sooner as it provides support and compression to help reduce pain and make moving around more comfortable. They are available in three styles to meet any stage of your surgery recovery.

HysterSisters

HysterSisters is a wonderful online resource that provides all kinds of information from diagnosis to recovery and beyond. They also provide

support for personal issues such as self-image and intimacy. And they carry a full line of helpful products, including cold packs and much more.

LYMPHEDEMA

Preventing Lymphedema

As covered in Chapter 7, lymphedema is fluid build-up that prevents the lymphatic system from operating properly. Your lymphatic system plays an essential role in your overall health. Here are some ways to help prevent lymphedema. Most of this section has been adapted from BreastCancer.org:

- Be aware of the early warning signs. Lymphedema can develop gradually and in stages. Some signs are tingling or numbness, achiness, puffiness or swelling, and/or a feeling of heaviness or tightness in your hand, arm, chest, breast, or underarm areas.
- Avoid doing too much too soon with the affected arm and shoulder. Generally, it's OK to start using them again for normal activities, like combing your hair, bathing, eating, and getting dressed.
- Be careful about lifting something heavy, for example, a grocery bag, gallon of milk, or a small child until you get a sense for what your arm can handle.
- Anything that involves repetitive use of your arm and upper body should be done with caution, for example, scrubbing, mopping, and raking. You should take frequent breaks and stop if your arm feels tired, heavy, or achy.
- Make sure any bras, camisoles, or tops you wear don't fit too tightly around your arms or chest.
- Don't allow the skin on your at-risk arm or hand to be pierced or pressured. Have bloodwork, injections, IVs, or blood pressure taken on the opposite side of where you had your lymph nodes removed or had radiation treatment. Or, if you've had

treatment on both sides, ask if you can have bloodwork or blood pressure measurements taken on another area of your body. Remind your care team about this at every appointment. You may want to buy a lymphedema medical alert bracelet, which can be found through the National Lymphedema Network.

- Be sure to ask a member of your health care team, ideally a trained lymphedema therapist, to figure out what types of exercise are best for you.

- You may want to consider a compression sleeve. These are stretchy garments worn on the arm to apply pressure that helps the flow of lymph up the limb. While experts don't agree on whether someone who hasn't had any lymphedema symptoms should wear a compression sleeve, some feel it's a good idea to wear one during physical and repetitive activities involving the arm, and while flying because of the change in air pressure.

Treating Lymphedema

With early detection, diagnosis, and the right treatment, you can manage lymphedema and prevent it from getting worse. Complete decongestive therapy (CDT), also called complex decongestive therapy, is considered the gold standard for treatment. It is a program that combines bandaging, compression garments, manual lymphatic drainage, exercise, and self-care.

Your lymphedema therapist can work with you over time to make sure your lymphedema stays under control, adjusting your plan as needed. For example, there may be times you need to wear a compression sleeve or other device around the clock, and others when you can get away with a few hours a day—or even skip a day or two.

Compression Sleeves

As mentioned above, compression sleeves can be worn to reduce the risk of lymphedema, as well as part of complete decongestive therapy.

It's never a good idea to buy a sleeve online or at a medical supply store without a proper fitting. Wearing the wrong type of sleeve may increase your risk of other problems.

Since my mission is to help make women feel beautiful, I've found a way to do so even with compression sleeves and gauntlets (fingerless fitted gloves). I've fallen in love with LympheDIVAs. LympheDIVAs turns these dull, medical-looking garments into fashion statements. With 100 stylish colors and patterns, the hardest part is which to choose. LympheDIVAs garments

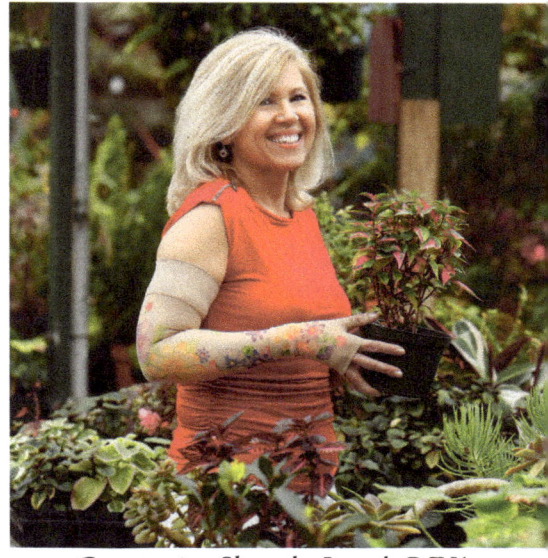

Compression Sleeve by LympheDIVAs

are regularly tested using a Vista-Medical FSA pressure mapping system to assure proper compression. Be sure to get assessed and measured by your health care team before buying one online.

HEAD AND NECK WEAR

If you're trying to conceal a visual scar in the neck region, choosing bulky jewelry, wearing a high neck or turtleneck sweater, or wearing fashionable hats or scarves are all great solutions. If you're really daring, there's always the option of camouflaging the scar with a beautiful tattoo.

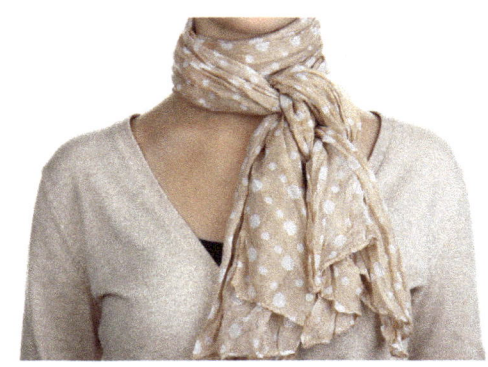

Neck scarf helps conceal scars

TATTOOING

Artistic and cosmetic tattoos can be the perfect alternative to reconstructive surgery.

You need to be finished with all cancer treatment and be completely healed before considering this option. Research to find the most reputable artist in your area.

Chest

Kelly's Story

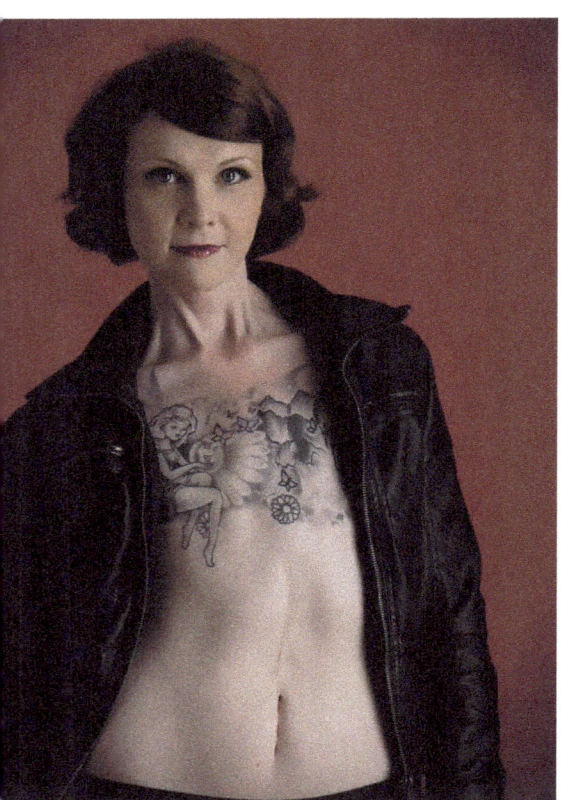

Kelly Davidson's beautiful tattoo art

I decided to tattoo my chest after my mastectomies because I wasn't interested in additional surgical procedures. For me, my breasts were not a definition of who I was as a woman. My tattoo represents things that I love: nature, things that are whimsical, and my favorite movie. The fairy represents me. The butterflies being released are the multiple cancers I have fought and won. In some sense, I went through a metamorphosis, breaking out of my cocoon, still the same woman on the inside but becoming something even more beautiful on the outside.

To find out more about Kelly, she shares her story in Chapter 11: Soul Sisters.

Stomach

Here's a beautiful image of a stomach tattoo. I've seen many different creative approaches to covering surgery scars. Try looking on Pinterest or Google Images to find some inspiration.

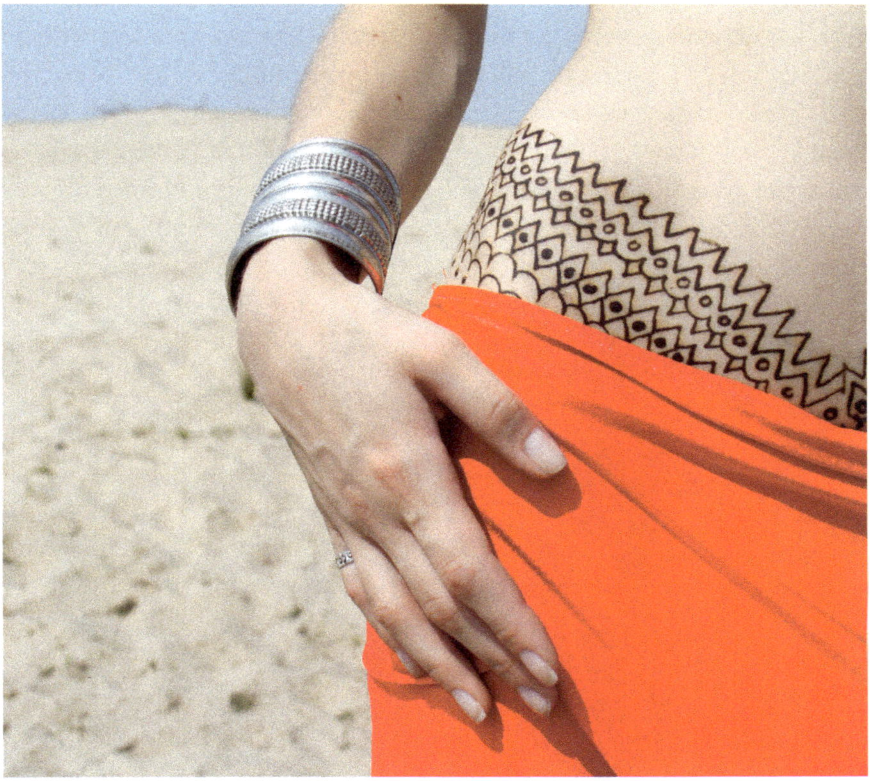

Stomach tattoo

Nipple and Areola

This is where a tattoo artist or plastic surgeon tattoos a nipple and areola in place. There are two options: a tattoo that is created by shadowing and coloring in the general area of the nipple, or a 3D version of a nipple tattoo that is more characteristic and life-like. The tattoo is completed in two phases (or more if need be) to create the detail, coloring, and specific characteristics of a real nipple.

If you choose to go to a tattoo artist, it's very important to find one who has experience working on reconstructed breasts. Your skin will be thinner, your breast tissue will be gone, your muscle will be stretched thin, plus you'll have an implant—a regular tattoo artist won't know that. If they tattoo at a normal depth, they may tattoo the muscle or puncture your implant, which will damage the implant and risk your health. Once you find a tattoo artist, ask to see photographs of tattoos they've done and be sure to ask questions, such as how many they've done and whether they're familiar with tattooing over breast implants.

Here Trish models her reconstructed breasts and nipple and areola tattoos.

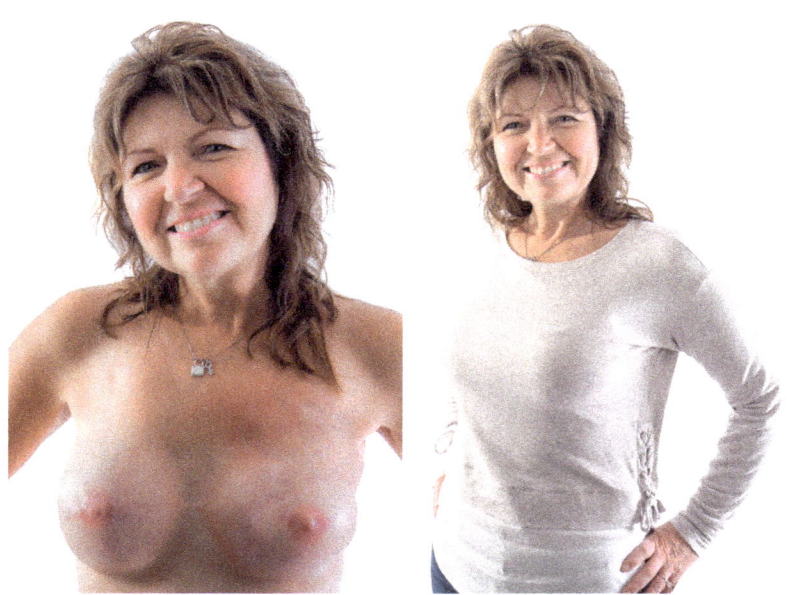

OTHER HELPFUL ITEMS

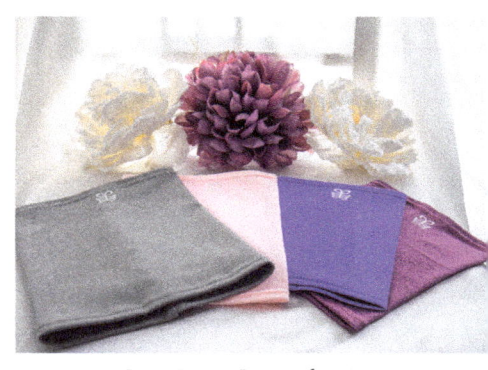

PICC Lines Covers

Peripherally Inserted Central Catheter (PICC) lines are a standard vehicle for administering chemotherapy. A flexible tube is inserted into a vein in your arm and will remain there for the duration of your treatment. In between treatments, the tube will be taped to your arm and covered with a dressing.

Picc Line Covers by Aya

Your cancer care facility should provide you with a cover to wear over the dressing. They will likely have a medical appearance and many will lose their shape shortly after wearing it, which causes the cover to shift and can be bothersome. Therefore, many women choose to wear a specialty PICC line cover. They come in a variety of beautiful colors and prints to match your wardrobe.

Lisa's Story

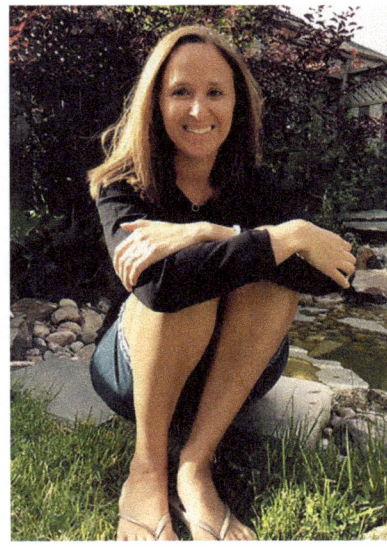

When I was diagnosed with cancer in 2006, part of the treatment process was receiving a PICC line. Throughout my treatment, I looked for something to cover it. That's when the idea for Aya Picc Line Covers came to me—fashionable and comfortable alternatives for patients undergoing cancer treatment. I wanted patients to proudly wear the Aya symbol, which represents endurance and provides them with strength on their journey. Today, with the help of my designer, Kirsty Gough, patients all over the world are benefiting from Aya Picc Line Covers.

(You can read more of Lisa's story in Chapter 11).

Seat Belt Cushions

If you are not a candidate for a PICC line, you'll likely have an implanted port, which is a disc that is placed under your skin in the chest area with a catheter between the port and vein. A port can quickly become sensitive, especially if something touches the area. A

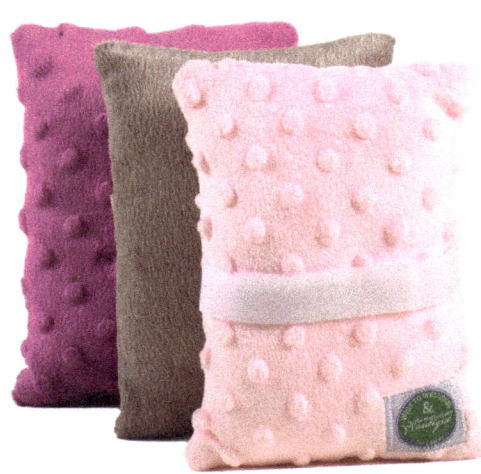

common complaint is seat belts. If this is a problem for you, seat belt cushions are a great way to provide comfort. They Velcro onto the belt strap and are adjustable according to your port placement.

Seat Belt Port Cushion

Donut Pillows

This little, round, hollowed-out pillow is good to use if you're having hemorrhoid pain as a side effect of chemo-induced constipation. Sit on a donut pillow if you have pain in your tailbone (coccyx), a common occurrence if you've been sitting in a recliner a lot after surgery. The donut hole allows the bottom of your spine to avoid pressure. Donut pillows are also good for hip pain and anal pain.

Breast Pillows

Breast pillows are very nice and comforting healing aids, as surgical incision sites can sometimes be bothersome. Breast pillows are soft, U-shaped pillows that rest under your armpit, making them great items to use while lounging

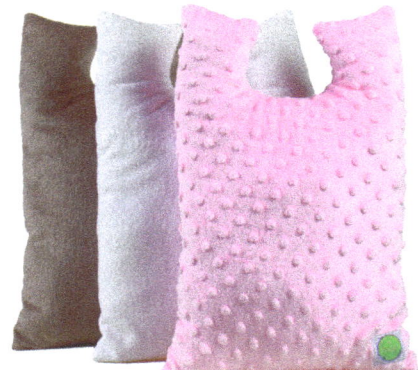

Underarm Breast Pillow

or sleeping. I've been told by many of my clients that this item is a must-have.

Wedge Pillows

If you've just come home from surgery and you must sleep on your back while managing surgical drains and dressings, a wedge pillow under your knees and lower legs elevates them. This flattens your spine and makes you more comfortable. Or place a wedge pillow under your head and shoulders to keep you from turning onto your side.

Post-Surgery Wear

The Brobe

The Brobe has hidden pockets for postoperative fluid drains and a detachable bra with front Velcro closure for easy wear. The three-quarter-length sleeves allow for easy IV access during treatment. The soft cotton blend fabric is comfortable and stylish.

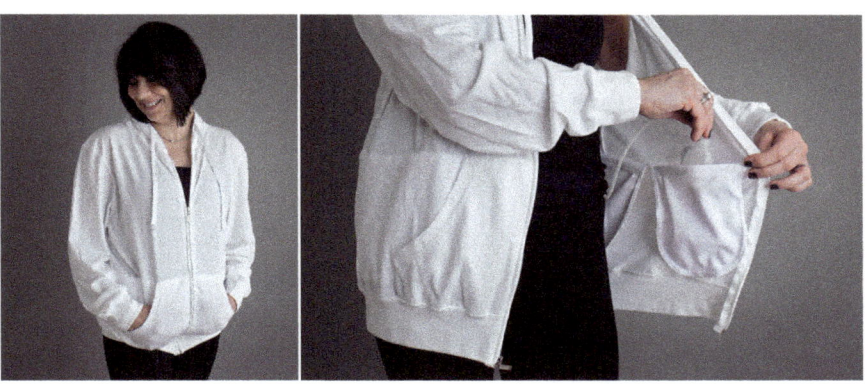

The Brobe (outside)   *The Brobe (inside)*

Reboundwear

Reboundwear is a stylish and comfortable post-surgical line of tops, jackets, pants, and hospital gowns, endorsed by medical professionals.

Night Sweats/Hot Flashes Sleepwear

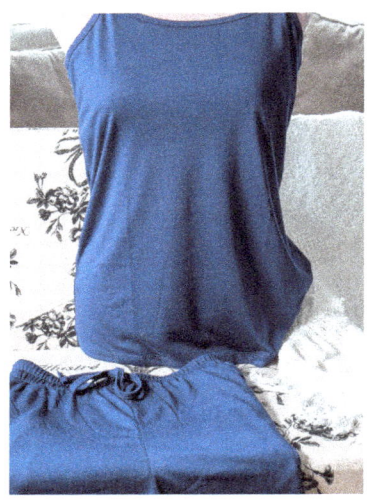

Cooljams offers proprietary sleepwear fabric that swiftly wicks heat and moisture and dries quickly.

Night Sweats Sleepwear by Cooljams

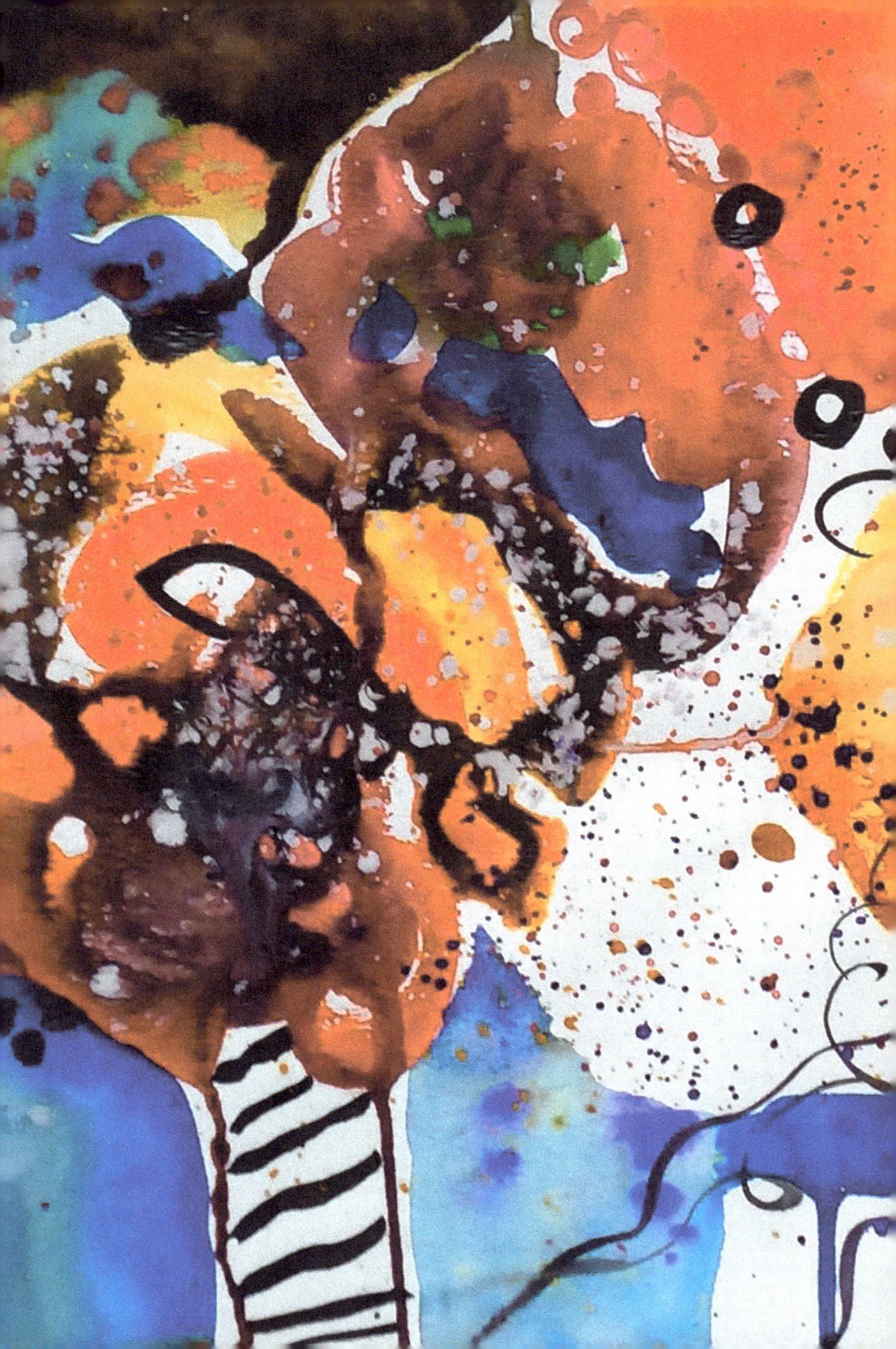

"I take very good care of myself—mostly because I didn't many years ago—and that served me well during chemo. Running every day made me feel calm and strong, even as my self-image suffered from my hair falling out."

—Edie Falco, television, film, and stage actress, breast cancer survivor

. . . .

9
Let's Get Physical

Embracing exercise and sex during treatment

EMBRACING EXERCISE

One of the goals I hope to achieve through *Healing Pretty* is to assure you that, even while undergoing cancer treatment, you can maintain a lifestyle close to what you are accustomed. If exercise was a part of your daily or weekly routine pre-cancer, in most cases, there is no reason why you should not be able to continue some form of physical activity while undergoing treatment. In fact, it's often recommended.

New guidelines released in October 2019 and published by the National Cancer Institute concluded that physical activity is beneficial for those living with and beyond cancer. Thirty minutes of aerobic activity, three times per week, is associated with improvements in physical function, quality of life, fatigue, depression, and anxiety. And, for people diagnosed with breast, colon, and prostate cancer, exercise is associated with longer life.

There are several factors involved when it comes to choosing your type and amount of exercise; for instance, what type of cancer you have,

your treatment plan, any pre- or post-surgical considerations, and your overall general health. Be sure to consult with your medical team and educate yourself on the risks involved before you start any exercise program. Let your medical team assess you and assist you in finding the best regimen for you.

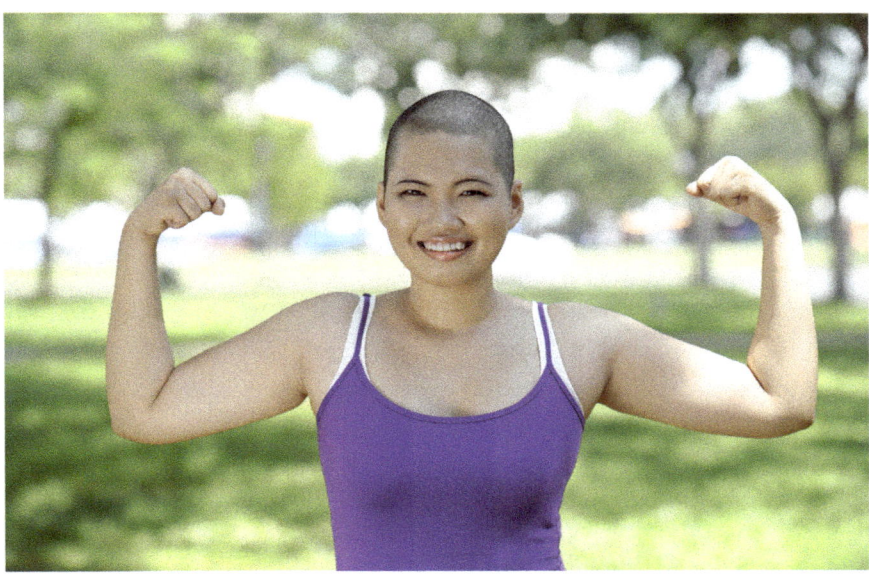

Before my experience working with women with cancer, I was under the impression that exercise would not play a part in treatment and recovery. I was wrong. Many of my clients are active, and even fit in regular workouts during treatment. Having the motivation to start is often the most difficult part, mainly due to fatigue. Once you're in the groove though, it's pure power!

You may not be able to keep up with your "normal" workout now, but there are many different types of exercise, each with their own unique benefits.

Exercise Options

....

"Having cancer does make you try to be better at everything you do and enjoy every moment. It changes you forever. But it can be a positive change."

—Jaclyn Smith, actress, model, dancer, businesswoman, author, breast cancer survivor

Walking and cycling are great ways to get moving and can also open doors for social opportunities. Yoga is another great option. Keeping yourself limber and balanced is crucial, while remaining mindful and aware of your body could be critical to getting you through tough treatments. Deep breathing and cultivating calm can help you feel better and make wiser decisions.

If you go to the gym, exercise with extreme care with regards to hygiene. Always sanitize weights and machines before and after use. You may want to consider wearing a surgical mask if you're comfortable doing so. Steer clear of public saunas and swimming pools, which may harbor bacteria. In addition, the chlorine in pools can burn sensitive radiation-treated skin.

If exercise is not an option for you, you can still practice some minor stretching, even if you're immobile. Rotating your arms and feet in circles can increase blood flow and keep joints and muscles flexible.

Exercise has many benefits, from keeping you limber and strong to improving your self-confidence. At a time when you may be feeling vulnerable, exercise will empower you to feel a sense of control.

YES TO SEX

For many of us, sexual intimacy is an integral part of our lives. I believe that if we are unable to maintain some level of intimacy, it has the potential to profoundly affect our self-esteem. Sex will likely be different than it was pre-cancer, but this need not be the end of it entirely.

Tips for Healthy and Safe Sex

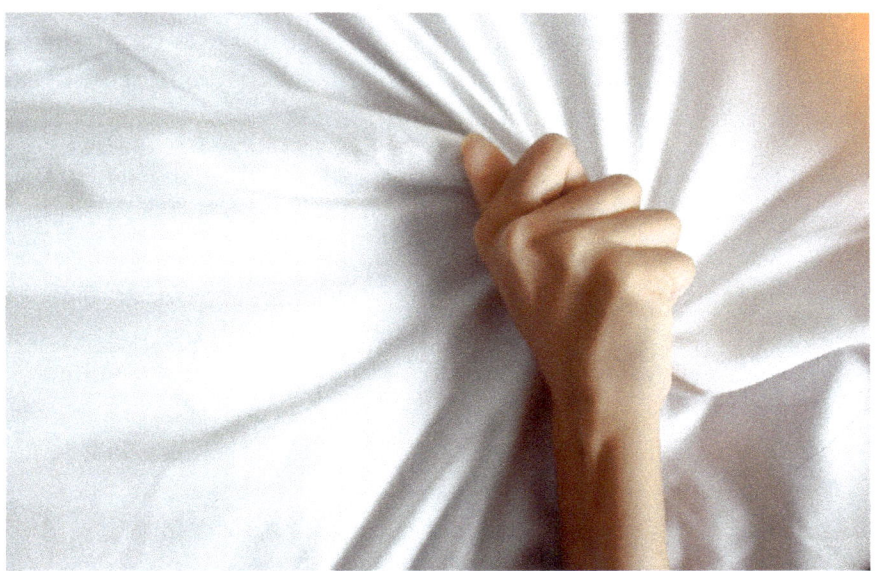

If you enjoy intercourse and hope to maintain a normal sex life, you should check with your medical team to make sure it's safe. If you have had any gynecological surgeries, you'll be advised to refrain from intercourse until you have your medical team's approval.

If you are concerned about becoming pregnant, be sure to ask about which methods of birth control would be best for you.

If you have a low white blood cell count or low platelet count below fifty thousand, it's advised to refrain from intercourse or using sex toys

that are inserted into the vagina. This is because there is an increased risk of infection or bleeding when your counts are low.

Chemotherapy can be excreted in vaginal secretions for 48 to 72 hours after a treatment. To be safe, wear a condom during sex until seven days after your last treatment to prevent your partner from being exposed to the chemotherapy drugs. If you have oral sex, use a condom.

It's not uncommon to experience pain during intercourse or penetration both during and after treatment. This is a result of vaginal dryness caused by inflammation, shrinking, and thinning of the vaginal tissue most often caused by lack of estrogen. Certain surgeries can lead to a shortened vagina, and radiation in the vaginal area can cause scarring. Here are some tips to help with comfort during sexual activity:

- Use a water-based vaginal lubricant during sexual activity, such as K-Y Jelly or Astroglide. There are quite a variety of lubricants out there and some contain fragrances, flavors, or herbal ingredients that you might want to stay away from, as they can be irritating. And don't use Vaseline or skin lotion as they can damage condoms and could raise the risk of yeast infection.
- For dryness, Replens Silky Smooth or K-Y SILKE-E are great vaginal moisturizers and are estrogen free. These should be applied 2–3 times a week, even if you're not sexually active as they help the vaginal tissue get back its natural moisture. And they can be used along with lubricants.
- You can find excellent organic vaginal moisturizers and lubricants made by a company called YES. Their products are formulated from plant extracts and contain only natural ingredients, certified organic by The Soil Association. Free from hormones, glycerine, parabens, and endocrine disruptors, they are safe to use to manage side effects of treatment for those with hormone sensitive conditions.
- To help with your estrogen levels, vaginal estrogens have been effective for some women. Be sure to discuss this with your

medical team—if you have a hormonally based tumor you may be advised to avoid these vaginal estrogens.

- If you've had radiation, some women have found that dilators help keep the vagina open and decrease scarring, making intercourse or penetration more comfortable. Again, be sure to discuss this with your medical team.

While many women can and do maintain an active sex life while undergoing cancer treatment (orgasms are still possible), it's also important to remember that you don't need to have intercourse to bond with your partner. Good, old-fashioned cuddling and caressing work just as well. This affection alone keeps the spark and intimacy alive until you're able to be sexually active again. Keeping the lines of communication open is important.

"Having cancer empowered me to take more risks. I knew beating cancer was going to shape me, but it wasn't going to be all of me."

—Hoda Kotb, television news anchor and host, author, breast cancer survivor

If you experience a lack of sexual desire, it could be a result of low self-esteem due to surgical scars or hair loss. Remember, you can always wear your wig and use wig tape to ensure it will stay in place during sex, or wear a sexy shirt if you're self-conscious about any surgical scars.

If you've had an ostomy, using an ostomy cover or camisole as camouflage can help with concerns that your partner may notice your bag.

Lastly, and most importantly, there is no reason to be afraid or embarrassed to discuss sexual issues with your medical team. They are there to care for your whole being and are happy to help you in any way they can. They have the experience and the expertise.

If you'd like to do a little exploring on your own, here are a few resources:

- Dr. Anne Katz is a renowned expert who provides information, education, and counseling to people with cancer and their partners about sexual changes during and after treatment. She has received numerous awards and has written a number of books.
- The American Cancer Society's *Sexuality for Women with Cancer*, NCI's *Self Image and Sexuality,* and Livestrong.org's *Female Sexual Health After Cancer*
- Professional societies can give you information about members in your area who have special training in sex therapy: The American Association of Sex Educators, Counselors, and Therapists (AASECT), and the National Association of Social Workers (NASW).

The links to these sites are included in the Resources Section (Appendix B).

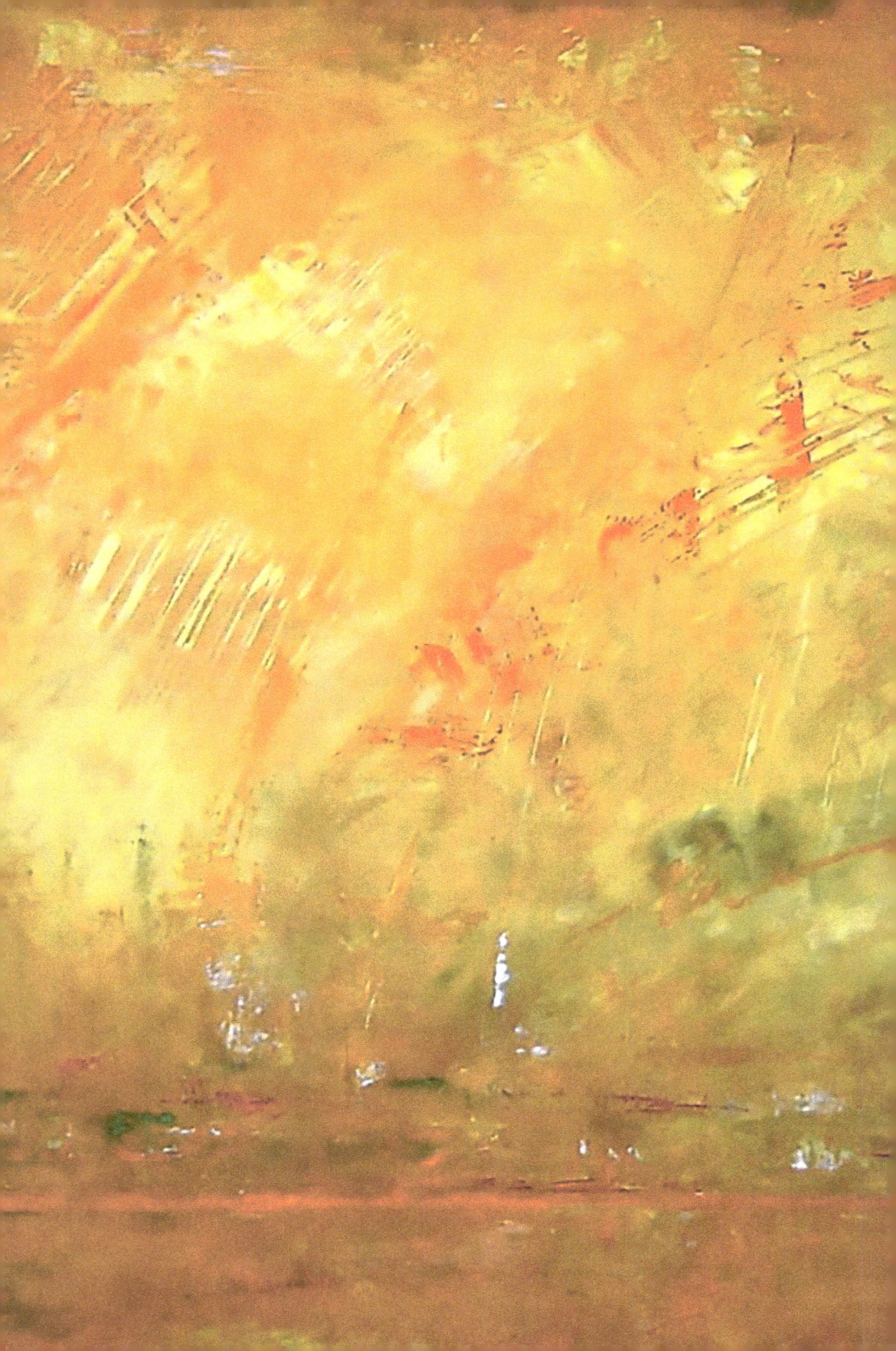

"Be grateful for each moment we have and be happy. But more than anything, live it fully."

—Valerie Harper, actress, author, 10-year lung cancer and leptomeningeal cancer warrior

. . . .

10
Brighter Days

Caring for you and your body after treatment

Throughout your treatment, your medical team has been by your side. Without realizing it at the time, they were providing a sense of safety, monitoring your every move. Then, treatment ends and many of my clients have described it as a relief and a time for celebration, but at the same time, they're scared to be on their own, having new questions and concerns.

Many cancer treatment centers offer programs to support you and your caregivers after treatment that include guidelines for managing your emotional, social, and physical health. There are also some great publications: The National Cancer Institute's *Facing Forward: Life After Cancer Treatment* and The Canadian Cancer Society's *Life After Cancer Treatment*. They can be found easily by googling them. I've taken some of their tips and shared them here, and added some from my clients.

Managing Your Feelings

Help take care of your emotions with these suggestions:

- Transform negative thoughts with yoga, meditation, or spiritual guiding. These mindful solutions may help to lessen or eliminate these feelings.

- Talk to survivors or read survivor stories. If you don't know anyone personally, there are local and online support groups who are always there to help.
- Talk to a professional therapist.
- Share your feelings with trusted friends and family.
- Laugh! It helps to counter stress and fear, and promotes a positive outlook. Watch a funny movie or try laughter yoga. (Yes, there really is such a thing!)
- Keep yourself busy with things *you* want to do. Pursue your hobbies, take a trip, live life to the fullest, do something you would never have done pre-cancer, follow your dreams.
- Volunteer: Helping others can take away your fears and could be very therapeutic and uplifting. Find something you're passionate about. You can walk, run, ride, or row for almost any type of cancer and cause. If you are able to, pick one or several events to get involved in. Your cancer care center or regional cancer society should be able to provide a list of causes.
- Perhaps you would like to become a *Healing Pretty* Soul Sister, sharing your story with other newly diagnosed women. If you would like to submit your story, I will include it in future publications or share it on my website at www.healingprettybook.com.

Healthy Lifestyle Changes

You can improve the way you look and feel by following some of these guidelines:

- Quit smoking
- Reduce your alcohol intake
- Exercise
- Eat organic fruits and vegetables
- Reduce salt intake
- Limit red meat
- Drink lots of water
- Add juicing to your daily regime

"I do feel different, but I can't quite articulate how. I've come out the other side of this, and I'm still not exactly sure how to define the difference, other than to say that I'm grateful, of course. But it's more than that. It's bigger."

—Julia Louis-Dreyfus, actress, breast cancer survivor

Many of the products we use today are loaded with chemicals and preservatives to make them last longer, smell pretty, lather more, and so on. From our grooming products to household cleaners, these items are likely to contain cancer-causing agents. Though it's nearly impossible to avoid chemicals completely, any attempt can help. You can start by using fragrance-free and non-aerosol products, and remember that good old-fashioned soap and water, vinegar, lemon juice, baking soda, and borax can be effective ways of eliminating many harmful chemicals in the home.

Your Appearance

In most cases, after treatment, your outward appearance will go back to the way it was before cancer. Your hair will grow, your eyelashes will come back, and your skin will rejuvenate. But in some cases, you may experience short, long-term, or permanent self-image issues caused by treatment or surgery. It can make recovery harder. Dealing with image issues can make you self-conscious, and it may affect your family, your social life, and your sex life. As mentioned in the book, most of these issues can be treated and camouflaged to help lift your self-esteem.

"I'm stronger than I thought I was. My favorite saying is 'This too shall pass.' I now understand it really well."

—Robin Roberts, television broadcaster, author, breast cancer survivor

Be prepared for comments or questions you may receive regarding your appearance. Some people won't know how to deal with it and could say the wrong things. Try not to take it personally—they mean well. Bring out the "funny in you" and come back with a witty answer.

Treat Yourself

Pamper yourself with whatever makes you feel good. Here are some ideas:

- A celebration wig
- Fun, colorful hats and scarves
- Make-up
- Lingerie
- Clothes
- Lipstick, lipstick, lipstick!
- Manicure
- Pedicure
- Massage
- Microblading
- Tattoo art to camouflage scars

I hope these ideas will help lift your spirits. Understand it's okay to mourn what you have lost, but always remember you are strong and you are a survivor.

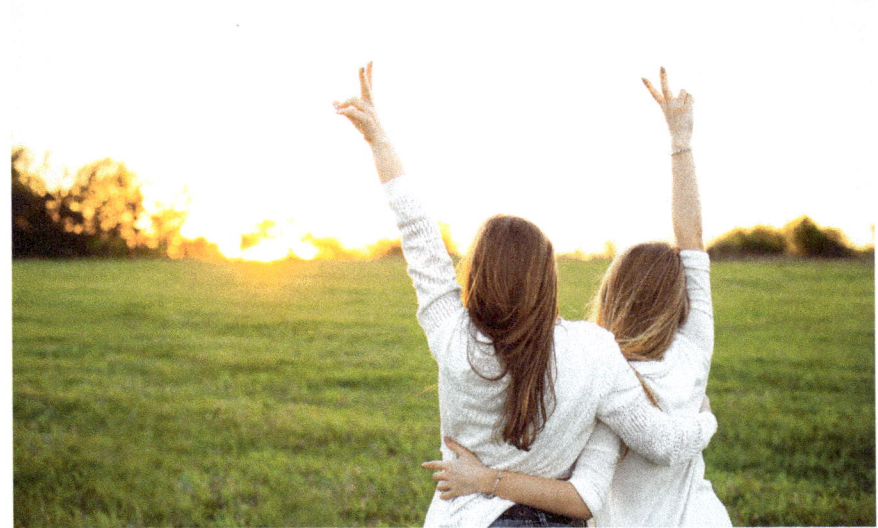

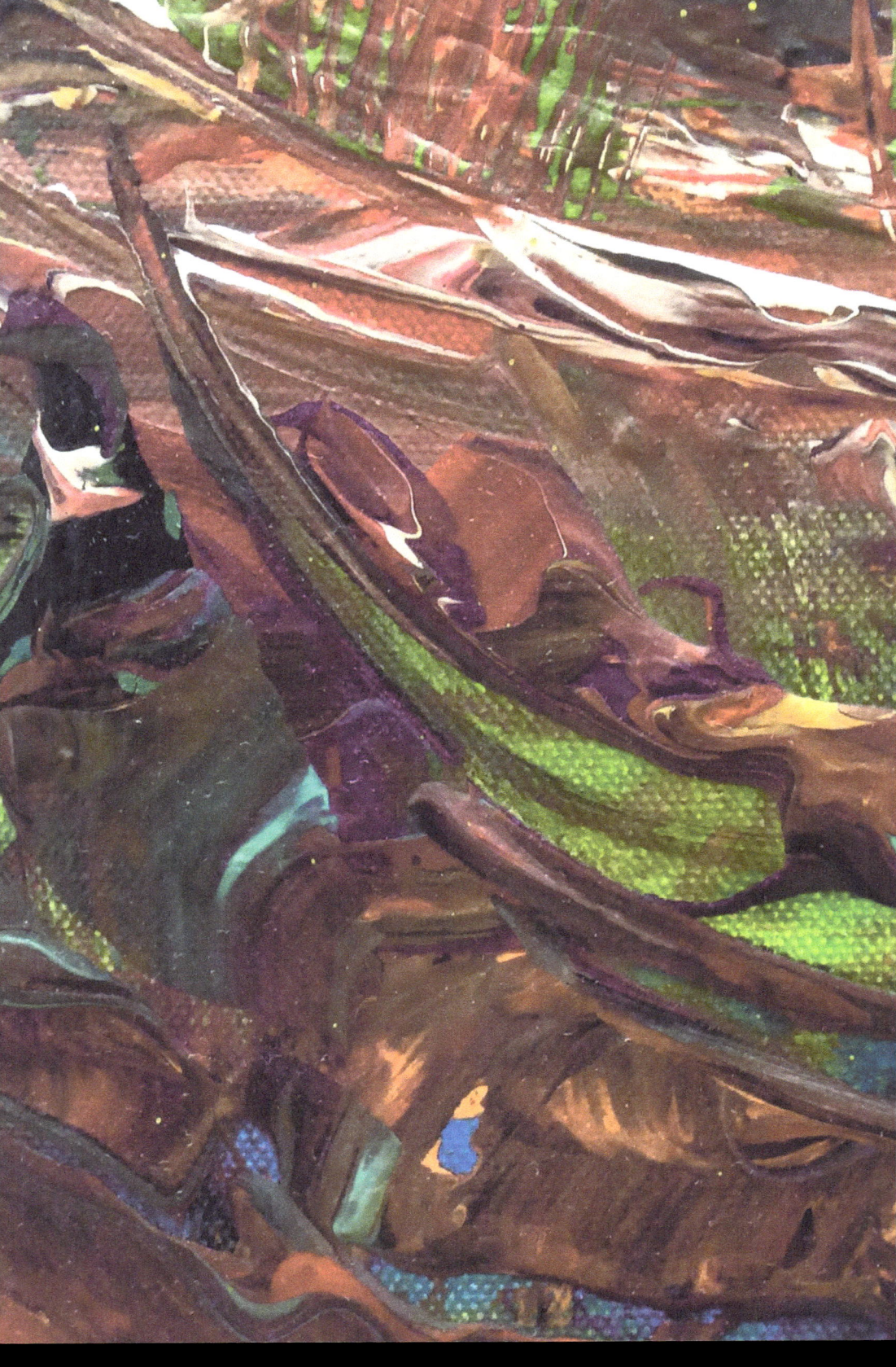

"The vanity was, I didn't want anyone to know. I didn't want the first thing they thought when they heard my name to be 'She has cancer, you know.' I didn't want my mother to know. I didn't want my daughter to know. I just didn't know how to deal with the feelings that were connected with having cancer. But then I thought, 'That's pretty arrogant. There's millions of women that have to deal with this every day. We have to work together. And it's my responsibility to help them.'"

—Diahann Carroll, *actress, singer, model, breast cancer survivor*

. . . .

11
Soul Sisters

*Personal stories and words of wisdom
from fellow cancer warriors*

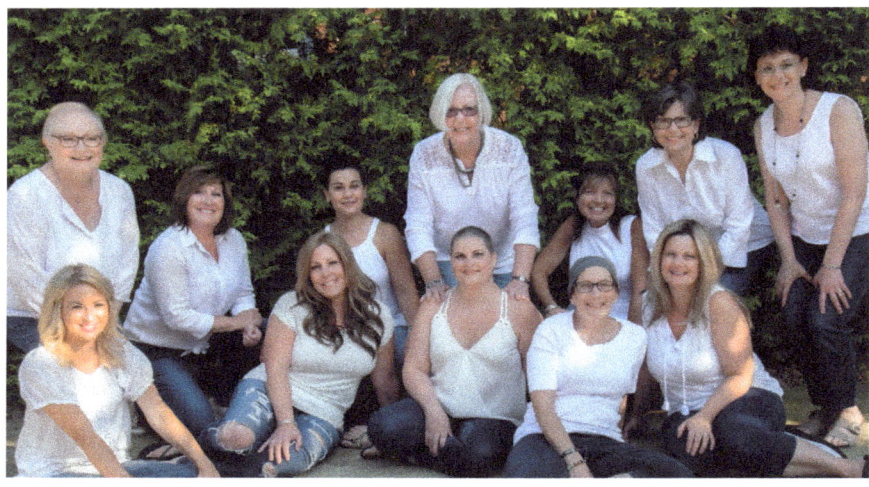

I'd like to proudly introduce you to my Soul Sisters, the authors of my final chapter. These women, my beautiful friends, have been where you are now, and they are eager to share with you what they've learned from their personal experiences, as well as the things that have helped them through it. Their hearts are huge, and their intentions are genuine. They've walked in your shoes, and they understand your struggles. Their generosity of spirit and openness of heart reinforce my belief in sisterhood. I have no doubt that their stories will inspire you as much as they have enlightened me.

Annette

Throughout my cancer journey, the one thing that stands out as having been the most helpful through it all was the support I've had. I'm blessed to have a family who never left my side throughout my entire fight—even when I may have wanted them to! I know some of you may not be as fortunate as I've been to have a big, supportive family, but I encourage you to reach out to anyone you can. There is always someone willing to help. Lean on your friends, go to support groups, talk to hospital volunteers. They all want to help. Don't do this alone!

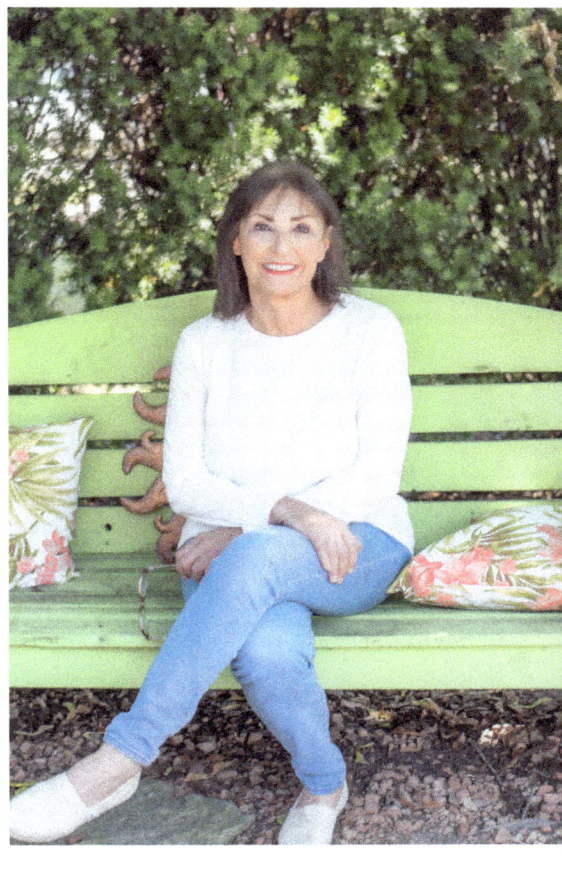

At one point, I had half a head of hair, as I refused to shave the other side. It was difficult for me to feel good about myself. I wasn't into wigs, so bandanas became my go-to look. But one day, I just really needed to feel like myself, so I plugged in my hot rollers (which was a daily ritual pre-cancer), rolled my half head of hair, and—voila! Not such a cute look, but it *did* make me feel better. The key is to do anything it takes to feel like yourself.

There are so many options and so much more information available to you now compared to what there was 16 years ago. The wigs are nicer, there are better products geared toward side effects, and those of you lucky enough to have Jackie are home free! I didn't have a "Jackie" when I went shopping for my first wig. I do have her as my little sis though, and I'm grateful for that.

Distractions are good, too. When I had cancer, Beanie Babies were the rage. My friends brought them to me when they came to visit. I BECAME OBSESSED! I started a collection. I think I ended up with over 100. It may seem trivial, but believe me, you want to keep yourself busy with whatever you can to take your mind off yourself for a while, even if it's something as silly as Beanie Babies. Go for it, but don't overextend yourself either. Get the rest your body needs.

Fight the fight. My doctor said I had a 15 percent survival rate, and 16 years later, I'm still here. You can do this, ladies. My prayers are with you.

Annette Apostol

Marcia

The kindness of strangers, medical staff, and volunteers touched me deeply, and I will be forever grateful.

Marcia Bear

Michele

The first few months of my breast cancer diagnosis were a blur, but I do remember feeling so very vulnerable and scared. Not knowing what is going to happen to you is terrifying. All the questions that really can't be answered. Questions like, what is my bald head going to look like? Am I going to have a nice round bald head, or am I going to find out I've some freakish bumpy bald head? What will I look like without eyelashes? We women love our eyelashes! What makes us feel better than a little mascara in the morning? Our eyelashes are what make our eyes pop, and let's face it: The longer and lusher they are, the more beautiful they make us feel. And WHAT!? No eyebrows either???? Eyebrows give our faces definition, and again, they help to bring out our eyes! I remember picturing myself as some grey-skinned alien. I had myself feeling ugly and depressed before I had even started any chemotherapy treatment.

I decided to cut my long blonde hair, preparing myself for what would eventually happen. I did not do it in steps. I cut my hair short and, to my surprise, I absolutely loved it! I felt beautiful, and when it did begin to fall out, I felt better prepared emotionally. There happened to be a make-up artist in the salon while I was there; she had some simple advice for me, the same tips for all her cancer clients: wear big jewelry, especially earrings, and bright lipstick with either a wig or a funky hat or beautiful colored scarves. I took her advice and went shopping for some beautiful costume jewelry, some brighter shades of lipstick, and cute hats and scarves. For some reason, I found I was not a wig person.

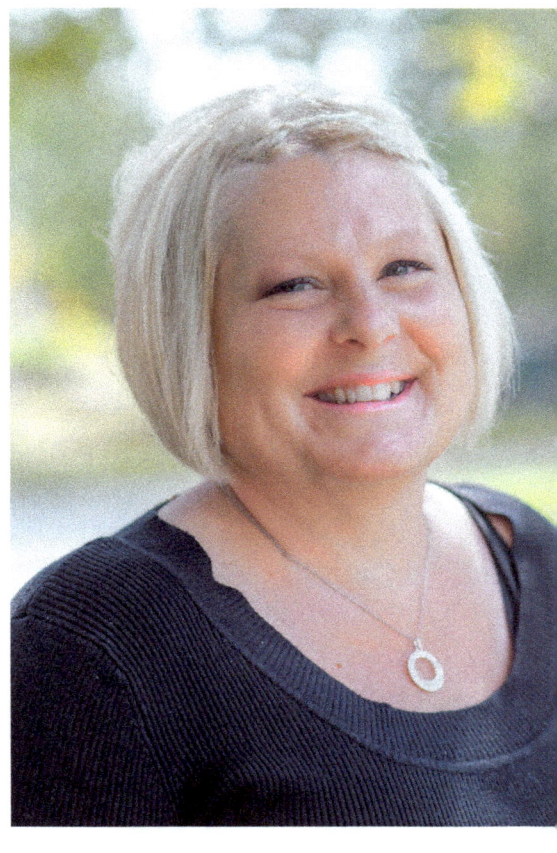

My last tip: moisturizer, moisturizer, moisturizer. Cancer and treatment do a number on the skin, drying it out terribly. A good facial cream and quality body moisturizer will do wonders for your skin during treatment. For me, it became a daily ritual, often more than once a day, to apply some relief to my skin.

And don't forget *water*. Drink lots and lots of water. We women should be doing that anyway, but especially during treatment; it's important to flush out the toxins. During chemo, I always drank a ton of water. Get that stuff out of your body and kidneys as quickly as possible.

To all the women out there recently diagnosed, remember you are not alone. Don't be afraid to reach out. Talk to women who have gone through this journey. They will be your biggest cheerleaders. Do your research. The web is full of information and answers to questions you may have—and you'll have questions.

When friends and family say, "Just call if you need anything," I suggest to DO IT! Call and let them know what you need. If your loved ones have not experienced cancer, then they have no way of knowing on their own. They want to help, but they need direction. Don't be afraid to give it to them.

My love and prayers to all the fighters.

Sincerely,

Michele Bosse

Trish

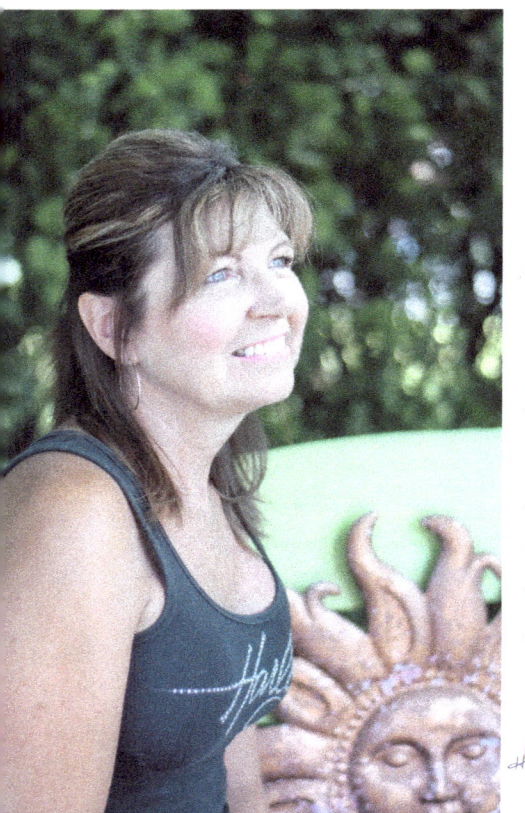

My best advice is to turn lemons into lemonade. From the beginning, I tried to have fun with a bad situation, bringing my friend Kim along to try on wigs. It was fun trying on different styles and colors knowing I'd not get that "one." I never had long, great hair—but now I could! Having a short wig and a long wig was fun. I posted pictures on Facebook and friends voted on which ones they liked (not that I asked them to!).

Then I had a head-shaving party. I made an easy dinner that included wine. All my friends took a turn shaving my head. We braided my hair, and Bob cut off my ponytail. The girls had fun gelling my hair into a Mohawk and then giving me a *Something About Mary* look before completely shaving it off.

My best friend, Patty, was my rock who brought me to my chemo treatments along with a few other friends. We posted pics on Facebook again!

After my diagnosis with breast cancer, I said that I wanted to take a vacation when I finished chemo. So I did! Patty and I went to Vegas and rented motorcycles with friends, and we rode to the Grand Canyon. I loved it.

I feel blessed to have Bob and some awesome friends and family who made this journey a little easier. Hope this story inspires someone else.

Trish Brookes

Sonia

OK, so now I have cancer—what am I going to do? I spent many sleepless nights wondering what would happen to me. I was on a rollercoaster ride (and by the way, I hate rollercoasters). This ride was going to twist and turn me around, and it was never going to stop.

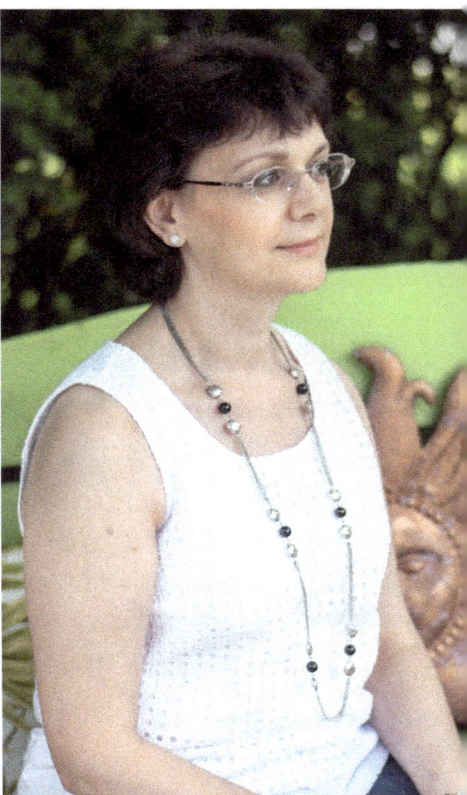

I've learned a great deal throughout my journey. I want to share some of those things in the hope that this advice will help others.

1. BE POSITIVE!

It's OK to cry and be upset. Then get ready to fight. One thing I learned the day I was told I had cancer is that your attitude has everything to do with survivorship. Remember: You have cancer, but it does NOT have you!

2. KEEP ORGANIZED!

With all kinds of appointments, pathology reports, blood work, and other information thrown at me, I was even more confused. Take a binder with dividers and organize everything. Ask for a copy of everything—each CT scan, bone scan, MRI, blood work, etc., and put it into your binder. Even though I can't understand very much on my pathology reports, I'm still happy to have them on hand. I even have a section at the beginning of my binder where I keep doctors' business cards and those of other professionals who have helped me through my journey. I also included an additional support section where I have contact information for my holistic nutritionist, chiropractor, massage therapist, naturopathic doctor, where I got my wigs and mastectomy bras, etc. Include a calendar where you can record all of your appointments. Now that I have everything in order, it makes it easier for me to look up my latest scans, surgery dates, appointments, etc. This helps me a great deal, and I carry my binder when I go to my appointments.

3. LEAN ON YOUR SUPPORT GROUP!

Don't go to any appointments alone. Ask family members or close friends to go with you. I found I could not understand or even take in what the doctors were saying. To me, all I heard was the "blah, blah, blah," just like the teacher in Charlie Brown. I took my entourage of support everywhere.

Appoint someone secretary and give them a notebook to record everything said during your appointment. This way, when you go home, you can read the notes and consult with your entourage so that you better understand what is going on. If I did not understand something, I'd highlight or record questions for my doctors in red ink.

4. TALK TO SURVIVORS!

These are the experts! Reach out to fellow cancer patients who have already gone through a similar journey. They have experienced chemotherapy or radiation treatments and can give you the best advice. Since I had breast cancer, I leaned on my fellow Pink Sisters. These ladies are the best people for me to talk to. I love the My Breast Cancer Sisters Facebook group, on which you're free to ask anything and your fellow Pink Sisters will give you honest opinions or advice. I also reached out to some family members and friends who have had breast cancer. They were an inspiration and an amazing support, especially during my chemotherapy treatments. People who have already been through it can offer you the best advice about what to do when you feel depressed or nauseous during chemo, or how to manage when your hair falls out. It's amazing how much easier your journey will be with their support. Don't be afraid to reach out to them. They will be more than happy to help you on your journey.

5. KEEP A JOURNAL OR DIARY!

I kept an inspirational journal. I wrote down uplifting poems, quotes, letters, and prayers. On days when I felt down and depressed, I turned to my journal to give me hope. Many friends would send me messages to cheer me up, and I'd paste those in my journal. It's awesome how a positive thought or message can completely change your mood.

6. HELP YOURSELF!

It's your journey, and only you know what is best for you! Listen to your body and follow your instincts. If something does not feel right, *act*. Do your research, ask questions, and seek advice from the experts. Don't sit there and wait for someone to drive the bus for you. It's *your* journey. You need to be the pilot. Even though I still go regularly to visit my oncologist at Karmanos Cancer Institute, I sought second opinions in the United States, just to make sure everyone was on the same page and that I was getting the best treatment possible. It gave me peace of mind.

7. TAKE CONTROL OF YOUR HEALTH!

Be willing to change your habits and lifestyle. I reached out to a holistic nutritionist, naturopathic doctor, massage therapist, and chiropractor. With their guidance, I made many positive changes in my life. I changed my diet and made better choices, switching to safer alternatives for a less toxic lifestyle. Don't be afraid to seek advice. Don't take something because the "experts" on Facebook recommend it. My naturopathic doctor provides me with adjunctive care. Using herbs and supplements and boosting your immune system can create a healthy and strong inner environment, one in which cancer won't be able to thrive. I feel good about the choices I'm making, and pray cancer stays away.

8. READ *Radical Remission: Surviving Cancer Against All Odds* by Dr. Kelly Turner

My daughter bought me this fantastic book when I was first diagnosed. This book summarizes Dr. Turner's research on how people around the world beat cancer without Western medicine, or after it has failed. She uncovers nine factors that can lead to a spontaneous remission—even after conventional medicine has failed. I found this book to be beneficial and began to implement some of the strategies that had worked for others in my own life. I highly recommend this book! It gave me an action plan and better armed me to fight my battle.

9. THE POWER OF MUSIC TO CHANGE ONE'S MOOD!

Sometimes, music is the only thing that gets your mind off things. My daughter made me a CD with some of my favorite inspirational music to lift me up when I felt down and depressed. I still remember the song "Don't Stop Believing" by Journey coming on the radio during one of my chemo treatments. I turned to the woman next to me and told her, "They're playing our song!" That song put a smile on our faces and put us both in a more positive mood. A friend gave me a CD filled with songs from our favorite teen heartthrob, Shaun Cassidy. My kids could not stand the music, but it made me happy. Listen to whatever

music makes you cheerful. Music has the power to bring you to a more peaceful place.

10. TRUST IN GOD!

My final and the best advice is to TRUST IN GOD! Having faith and a positive attitude is what pulled me through. When I was at my lowest, I got down on my knees and prayed. I found comfort and guidance in reading scripture. "Leave all your worries with Him, because He cares for you" (1 Peter 5:7). I learned to take something negative—my cancer and all the suffering it brings—and to offer it to God to turn into something good. "The Lord is my strength and my shield; my heart trusts in Him, and He helps me" (Psalm 28:7). My faith has grown, and through my illness, my relationship with God has become stronger. When I prayed to Him, He always guided me to make the right choice.

I want to thank Jackie Apostol-Pizzuti from Wigs to Wellness for giving me the opportunity to share what I've learned throughout my cancer journey. I wish *Healing Pretty* had been available when I was first diagnosed. I'm sure newly diagnosed cancer patients will find it a beneficial and comforting resource.

God bless you all! I wish you much joy, love, and good health!

Sonia Coletti

Daniella

My name is Daniella Czudner. I'm a 42-year-old wife, mother, and high-school English teacher. Until recently, I was one of the healthiest people I knew. My clean lifestyle has always included a balance of healthy eating, yoga, strength and cardio training, and plenty of fun with family and friends. However, all of this changed on April 29th, 2013, when a very large tumor was discovered on my right ovary via ultrasound.

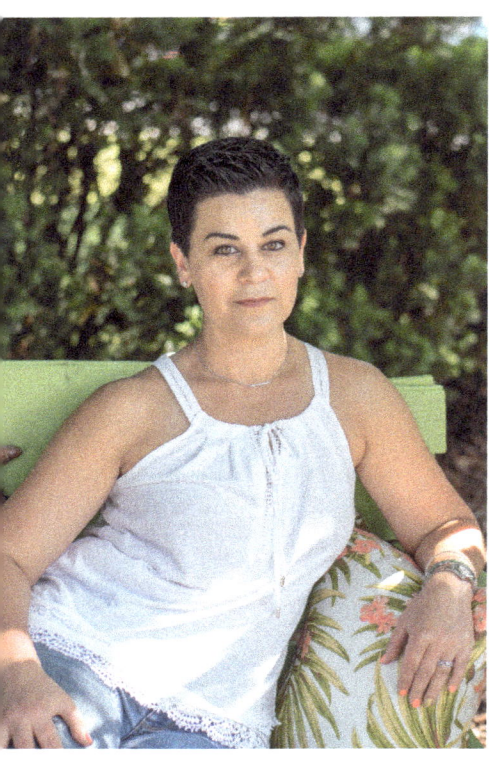

Once I allowed myself to accept the truth that I could not change, I prepared myself for six rounds of chemotherapy. My oncologist ordered a combination of Carbo and Taxol, chemo treatments that I could receive in my home rather than at the hospital, where I had had surgery. I was ready for the worst and prepared my children for what I thought was going to be the worst four months of their lives. Our approach to cancer was the same as our approach to every topic—tell the truth. After all, at 10 and 12, if we did not tell the truth, they would figure it out. It allowed them to feel there was no reason to be afraid. They both felt this was a challenge, but they never feared the disease would kill me. In the end, my family allowed me to set the tone for dealing with cancer. I did so with a little bit of humor and a whole lot of living. When my hair started to fall out, I cried for two days and then planned a party. I gathered my family and close friends, ordered a teal velvet cake shaped like clippers, and the kids took turns cutting and clipping. I took control and removed the fear and sadness for those who cared most.

My tolerance for chemo was remarkable and, although I lost my hair, suffered from the usual aches and pains, and endured the famous "chemo brain" that left me in a fog some days, our life as a family continued as normal. It meant soccer and football, birthdays and barbeques. In fact, in many ways, we were enriched by the diagnosis. Life slowed down, and I could reconnect with people and hobbies that were simply pushed aside because of the busy-ness of life.

To be physically prepared for the side effects of chemo, I focused on eating a mostly plant-based diet and made sure that I either walked five kilometers or did yoga every day. I think there are some obvious physical benefits to this, but the psychological benefits were what saved me. I've now gone back to teaching, a job I love. I've found purpose in fundraising at my local Cancer Centre and speaking to as many people as I can about ovarian cancer, its symptoms, and the need for women of all ages to be more aware of their bodies.

I'm currently back teaching full time, enjoying yoga and some good ol' fashioned cardio with weight training. I'm also very active in many fundraising and cancer awareness initiatives. Life 2.0 is amazing.

Daniella Czudner

Kelly

Never stop laughing and smiling. Keep family close by, because they will be the ones to always be there for you. My mom, aunt, and cousin shaved their heads with me before I started chemo, participated in numerous cancer events—even dressing up like Care Bears and Smurfs for Relay for Life—and always gave me hope that I'd beat cancer, all three times.

Most of all, never give up. It will be hard at times. You may feel alone, sad, and angry; but just look around at everything you must fight and everything you must live for, and know you are not alone, and you'll kick cancer's ass. There was something that I said once in an interview when I was 11-years-old that still sticks with me: "Don't think of cancer as a bad thing or giving up. Just keep going with your LIFE."

Kelly Davidson

Jen

Imagine finding out that your mother has cancer, and only five months later, finding out that you'll be fighting it as well. At the age of 31, I

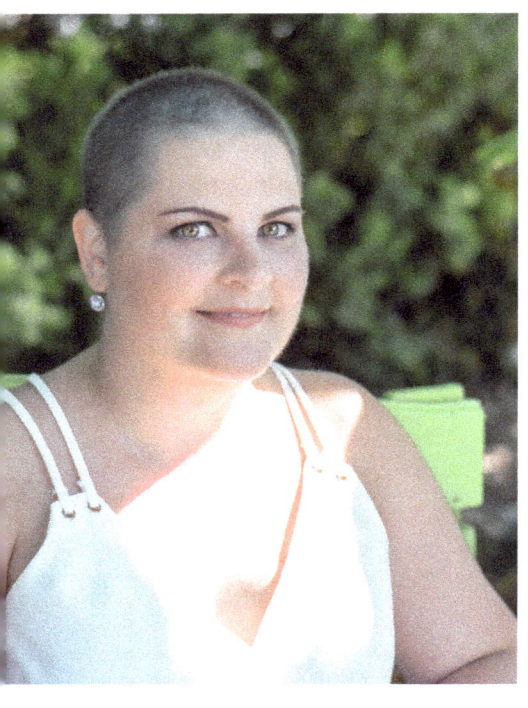

was diagnosed with ductal carcinoma triple-negative breast cancer, stage 2B. I've had a double lumpectomy, eight rounds of chemo, and a bilateral mastectomy with immediate reconstruction at this point.

Cancer is ugly; it's raw, you're lost and numb with fear, chaos, and uncertainties. You begin to appreciate the little moments, like having a bit more energy one day, and moments when you can try and enjoy your child's laughter. Find your reason to fight; for me, it was my son. I just could not imagine missing out on his baseball games and losing his first tooth. He is my strength and my reason to live.

It's so very hard, but try to stay positive. There will be many moments of difficulty and despair, but rely on the three *F*'s to pull you through: Faith, Family, and Friends.

In your deepest and darkest moments, remember to "just breathe."

"I survived because the fire inside me burned brighter than the fire around me."—*Joshua Graham*

Jen Ellwood

Lynda

I hear the words, but not really. My mind takes me to another place—anywhere but here—the loose button on my shirt, the errands that need to be done, the crinkly feel of the paper on the examining table in the doctor's office. I am only 48 years old, but tests confirm invasive breast cancer and further treatment is required—chemotherapy, radiation, and Herceptin treatments.

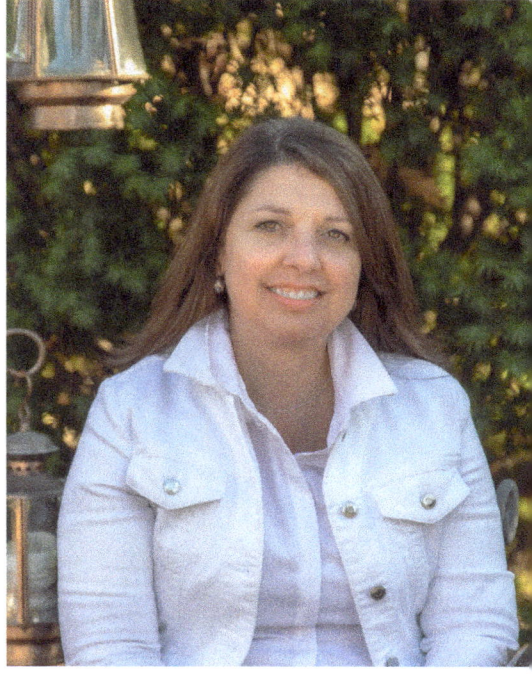

Everyone in the cancer clinic is helpful, thoughtful, and compassionate, but the information provided can be overwhelming in the beginning. A fellow patient who can see my apprehension and distress approaches me and gives me very good advice. He advises me that, no matter what, I would be in control of my treatment and to not lose myself in all that was to occur in the coming months, because I should stay true to who I was. It is in that moment that I decide that having cancer—and its related debilitating treatment—would not define me or take over my life. I discuss this with my children, and we agree that the next day would be business as usual—work for me and school for them.

I am a CPA and the CFO of an innovative manufacturing company with many diverse responsibilities, and my colleagues are supportive of my decision to continue working through treatment. It is not easy—I work Monday through Thursday and have chemotherapy treatments on Friday. The weekends are for regaining my strength. The cancer clinic has wonderful therapists, and they help to guide me through the process and to stay focused. Of course, it is not easy to hide the effects of treatment, including hair loss, but wigs, caps, and scarves help.

There will be times when you'll want to take a step back—this may be a day or a week—and grieve the loss of the life you once led. But know that this is okay; it is part of your success story and a mark of your progress. While it can be monumental in the beginning, the key for me was to have small goals: Get through this one day, this one week, this one month, and soon you are celebrating the end of treatment.

Immerse yourself in the love and support of your family, friends, co-workers, and medical professionals. Together, you will form a team; accept their kindness, guidance, and willingness to aid. Rejoice in each step successfully taken, and do not be afraid to ask for help or a shoulder to cry on. Ultimately, know that each journey is different and unique, and we are all survivors.

Stay in control, remember who you are, stay true to you—be the leader of your own story.

Lynda Dettinger

Karin

I'll always be grateful that my hairdresser said to pick out my wig before I lost my hair. She was so right. She also suggested bringing friends along. "Face it, husbands aren't always the best judges!" she said.

The next thing is to find a great person who sells wigs, and that person would be Jackie! Go to the Look Good Feel Better workshop as early as you can. You may think you won't use all that make-up, especially if you're like me and did not wear a lot to begin with, but you likely will, eventually. Wearing make-up when you don't feel good and look worse *does* help! I was also grateful that my oncologist told me exactly when my hair would fall out, so I was ready. She was right, down to the day!

One thing that made my heart sing was how my friends organized meals delivered to our house on my chemo days. That was helpful. I did not ask them to do this. They just did it. They also drove me to Windsor for chemo since it was too difficult for my husband to accompany me, as a cancer survivor himself.

I went out for lunch with a couple of friends every other week, which made me get dressed, put on make-up, see people and laugh, all of which made me feel less ill.

Karin Forshaw

Deb

What made my experience on this journey was my family and friends—and some people I did not even know—standing strong with me, making me feel beautiful inside and out just by the chats, hugs, and mainly, the visits. I never felt alone, ever. My journey was their journey. My belief in God and prayer was also comforting, as was my daily cup of green tea.

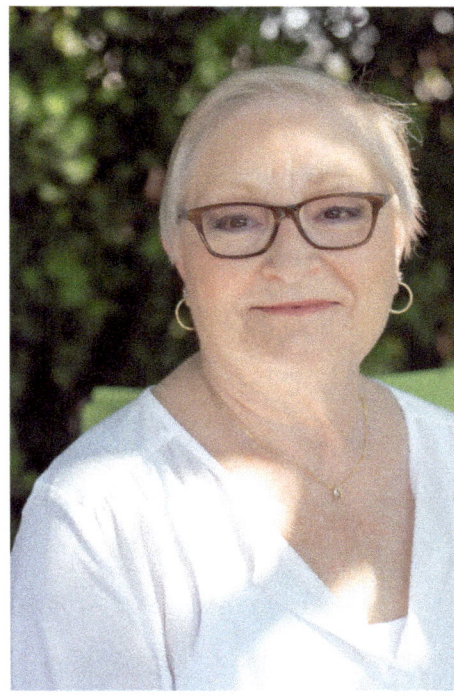

I returned to work ten months later to people I regarded as a family and had missed dearly. I started eating healthier and walking as regularly as possible.

But mostly, I think of that final day when I whacked that gong and decided that this is my re- birth, and I deserved it.

God Bless,

Deb Kokovai

Sandra

In July of 2015, I was diagnosed with breast cancer. It was in the nipple of my left breast and one lymph node. I was shocked and devastated. I had chemo to shrink the tumor, a double mastectomy, radiation, and Herceptin.

From the very beginning, I knew I was going to fight this. I wanted to live! I still had things I wanted to do and accomplish.

What got me through the tough times was my family and friends. They encouraged me and were always around me. I've three grandchildren who love their grandma. I was determined to be here for them.

My daughter-in-law was pregnant with their first baby, so during the tough times, I knew I wanted to be here when he was born and for him to know me. He gave me the strength to fight.

I cut out articles from the paper about people who were fighting cancer and beating the odds. They were my inspirational stories.

I had quotes all over the house. Here are some of my favorites:

HOPE

Hope is putting faith to work when doubting would be easier.

FAITH

Faith is where you close your eyes and open your heart, moving beyond the familiar and embracing the unknown.

ACCEPTANCE

Accept what is, let go of what was, have faith in what will be.

The book *Healing Is a Journey* helped me, too. Jackie from Wigs to Wellness always made me feel better. Her wigs helped me so much when I first lost my hair, and the Look Good Feel Better group was so uplifting.

Finally, my faith played a big role in my recovery. I believe that God gives us the strength to get through tough times.

Sandra Kavanaugh

Kelly

It was November 2016, when I was told the words you never want to hear: *You have breast cancer.* I was devastated. Very soon after being diagnosed, my beautiful neighbor came over for a visit and gave me an awesome, well-written book called *Healing Pretty*. This book not only had real life stories about women sharing their experiences while going through cancer, but it showed me what I might expect or go

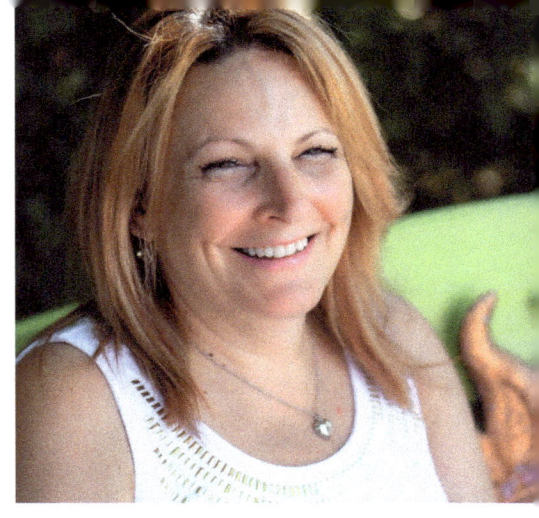

through myself. While reading this book, it gave me such a good feeling, and some strength to know that I'm not alone anymore.

Stay positive and surround yourself with your family and friends.

God bless! Love ya!

Kelly Kime

Jill

You are the strongest when you are the most vulnerable. Little did I know how strong I was until I was diagnosed with breast cancer at the young age of 23. Though at the time I felt like my entire world had come to a halt, I'm proud to say that seven years later, I'm a CANCER CONQUEROR!

Keeping a positive mindset helped me to find humor in my cancer journey. I like to break it down into three parts—the three *B*'s: Boobs, Balding, and Blogging.

BOOBS

After having a prophylactic double mastectomy, I developed the motto: "No Cancer, New Boobs." My mission was to take back what cancer took from me, and I must say, I got back even more. While the boob mission was long and enduring, my new breasts have given me more self-confidence, along with a whole new wardrobe.

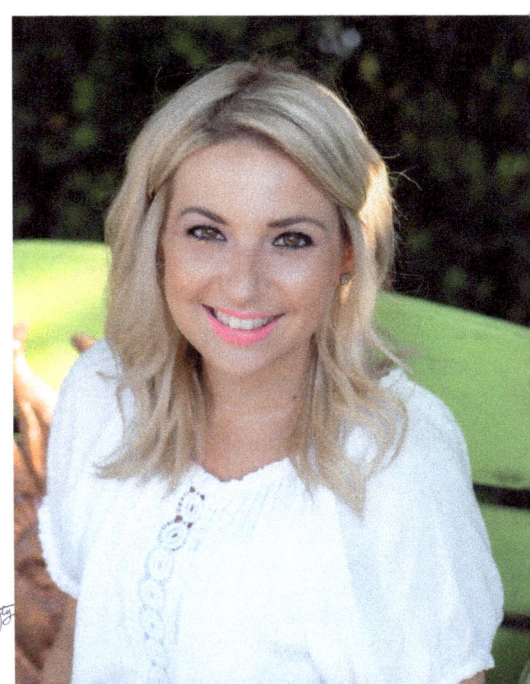

BALDING

As odd as it sounds, I found great satisfaction with pulling chunks of hair out of my head. It was liberating, and it felt like a symbol for what I was going through. I felt like a warrior. On top of it, I got a Mercedes—no, not the car—a blonde bombshell wig. Mercedes was a fancy girl, and I only took her out for special occasions.

BLOGGING

Keeping an online journal was a great place for me to reflect on my journey, and it also helped others understand what I was going through without having to call me multiple times a day to see how I was feeling. In turn, it became a comic relief for me to write about all the silly things I did in the cancer clinic while under the influence of strong medications.

My advice for any new cancer survivor is to *find balance*. What might work for one survivor may not always work for another. Treatment affects every one of us differently. Don't be afraid to be "selfish" and ask for help. Trust me; people want to help you. Lastly, always remember that there is life after cancer, and it's even more beautiful than before.

Jillianne Laframboise

Darlene

The best thing that I did to help myself feel pretty after losing my hair was to get a wig that looked almost exactly like my hair. Jackie picked it out for me, and it was perfect! The color was very close, and she cut it in a similar style. Even people who knew what I was going through could not tell I had lost my hair or that I was wearing a wig! It helped me to feel confident about going out in public, and once I went back to work, I wore it every day and felt good about it.

Another great thing was going shopping with my teenage daughter before I lost my hair and buying a bunch of pretty scarves together. It was a great bonding moment for the two of us, and the scarves helped

me deal with my baldness without having to wear my wig all the time. I mostly wore them around the house and when visiting the cancer clinic for my chemo treatments, etc. I even wore them to bed, as they kept my head warm at night.

There were many women whom I'd talked to who had gone through chemo and hair loss. Talking to these women helped me cope with my hair loss, as they were all so supportive and caring, and it helped to see their confidence and knowing that I was not alone.

Darlene Kopacz

Sue

In September 2011, I was diagnosed with breast cancer that had already spread to my liver and bones. For this reason, I did not have a mastectomy. I wouldn't have benefited from it.

I was given six months, give or take two months, depending on how strong I was. My abdomen was full of fluid. I was drained of a gallon the first time, and kept going back to the ER every few days to get drained, until they put a drainage tube in me so I could do it myself at home every other day. That went on for a few months, until the tube got infected and I ended up in the hospital on IV antibiotics for a week.

I started chemo on October 14, 2011. I wasn't going to do chemo because, being a nurse, I had seen too many patients who had suffered from the side effects and died anyway. One of my other doctors talked me into it. He said to try it. "If it does not help," he said, "and you don't like it, you can always quit." So I did try. And I responded well. The spots on my liver shrunk to almost nothing, the fluid in my abdomen disappeared, and the spots on my bones disappeared. I became stronger and could return to work in November 2012. I used my personal experience to help my patients with cancer.

I had a routine CAT scan in January of this year, and it showed cancer had returned to my abdomen, with spots on my liver and around the bowel. So I started chemo again on February 25. The last scan I had last week showed that the chemo is working.

I've learned that how many days you have left is not as important as making the most of every day. Do what you like. Do what makes you happy. Laugh a lot. Life is too short to be miserable.

Make yourself look good. Wear make-up every day, even if you're not going anywhere. Then when you look in the mirror, you'll make yourself happy.

Hair loss was no big deal to me. I did not have very nice hair to begin with. Taking a shower is so fast now that I don't have to bother with shampoo and conditioner, or shaving my legs. Put your make-up on, grab your wig, and go!

Most importantly, stay positive!

Sue Litster

Tanya

I was 41 when I was diagnosed with breast cancer. I thought my life was over. I did not know anyone my age who had breast cancer. I thought I was going to die. To make matters worse, I went on the Internet and researched breast cancer. I went on scary sites about women who were dying of breast cancer. I was on the Internet 24/7, and I became very depressed. I realized I had to stop going on the Internet.

I ended up meeting a lady who worked with my husband who was ten years cancer-free. Then I met another woman who was a 17-year survivor. Any time my mind would go to a bad place, I'd think of these women.

Here is what I learned: Stay off the computer! There are so many cancer survivors that we don't know about—because they are busy living

their lives! Find a support group. It helped me to know other survivors who are many years out of treatment and cancer-free.

Stay away from negative people and surround yourself with positive ones. I kept my diagnosis from a lot of people—some people just say the stupidest things.

Invest in a good wig. I always left the house in my wig. I'd wear hats or headbands on top of them. No one knew I was wearing it. I did not want people staring at me. That's why I always wore my wig.

When washing your face, don't touch the eye area and eyebrows. If you don't touch them, I found the hair won't fall out as quickly.

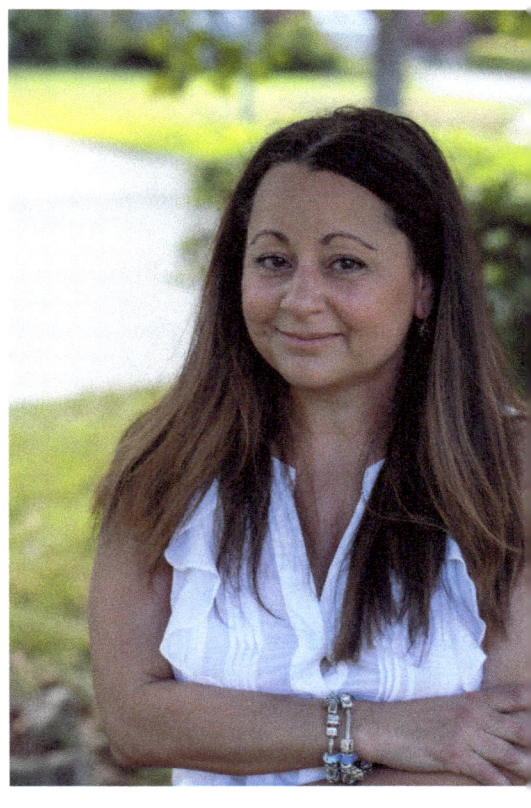

My hair started falling out after my second chemo. The best thing that I did was shave my head. It was torture to watch my hair fall out slowly.

Eat lots of fiber! I had bad constipation. The doctor gave me all kinds of meds, but the only thing that helped was lots of bran cereal and plenty of water.

Drink lots of water, especially after chemo, to flush out the toxins.

I was on Taxol. To prevent bone pain, I took Claritin the day before chemo and for a couple of days after (be sure to check with your doctor before you do this).

Treat yourself after each chemo. I'd buy lipstick at the Mac counter the day after chemo. It's something to look forward to, because you deserve it!

Plan a little trip when you are done. Something else to look forward to!

Sign up for the Look Good Feel Better program! They provide lots of great information, plus a box of free make-up!

During radiation, get cream to prevent burns. The doctor gave it to me. I did not burn while I was going through treatment, but I burned in different areas up to a month after it was over.

Keep busy!

Always remember, you can do this! You're stronger than you think!

Tanya Marra

Kathy

It started with the dreadful news of being told I needed a double mastectomy followed by chemotherapy. My husband, Emerson, and my daughter, Lori, would give me my Neulasta shots in my stomach (chemo booster). Ladies, if you must do this, I found taking a Claritin helped with nausea and bone pain. During chemo, I wore cold gloves, which the cancer center provided. It truly helps your fingernails from lifting. And get lip cream. You'll need it.

Then, of course, came the hair loss. The first wig salon I went in to, I was humiliated—but then my husband found Jackie. The woman is my rock. She fixed me up and gave me back my dignity. It was the first time I'd laughed in months. After that, I went back for other products. I opted for reconstructive surgery, starting with expanders, but until the process was complete, I wore breast prostheses.

Try and get a good amount of sleep. Propping yourself up works wonders.

If it upsets you that you think your girlfriends are ignoring you, call them! Ask them to go to chemo with you. You'd be surprised by how involved they want to be—but they're scared.

Cancer wears you down. But you CAN overcome it. If you need to cry, *cry*. Whether you're alone or you have another's shoulder, it works. Take a bubble bath. Listen to music. Put on your favorite lipstick. Throw on your wig and visit people. There is a light at the end of the tunnel, and the light will get closer every day.

Have faith, be strong, and stay positive. Live, Love, Laugh.

Kathy McIntyre

Rona

From the moment I was diagnosed with Non-Hodgkin's Lymphoma, which seemed to come out of nowhere, everything moved fast. I suggest a journal to write down everything that happens in your day, even if it seems unimportant.

I also suggest exercising from the very beginning of treatment. You won't want to, but try to get up and just move around and stretch. Very short walks. Light hand weights. Anything to keep the muscles strong and the blood moving.

Ask your doctor lots of questions so that you understand everything and can write it in your journal.

Join a support group if you can find one.

Try massage and acupuncture for aches and pains, but ask your doctor first if it's allowed during treatment.

Be sure to drink a lot of water.

Make sure you tell your friends and close family exactly how you feel so that they know what's going on. Don't be afraid to say you just aren't feeling well.

Don't worry about groceries, cooking, housework, or laundry. And lastly, get as much sleep as you can.

Also, I thank Jackie. My experience would have been so much harder without her advice and expertise.

Rona Paquette

Peggy

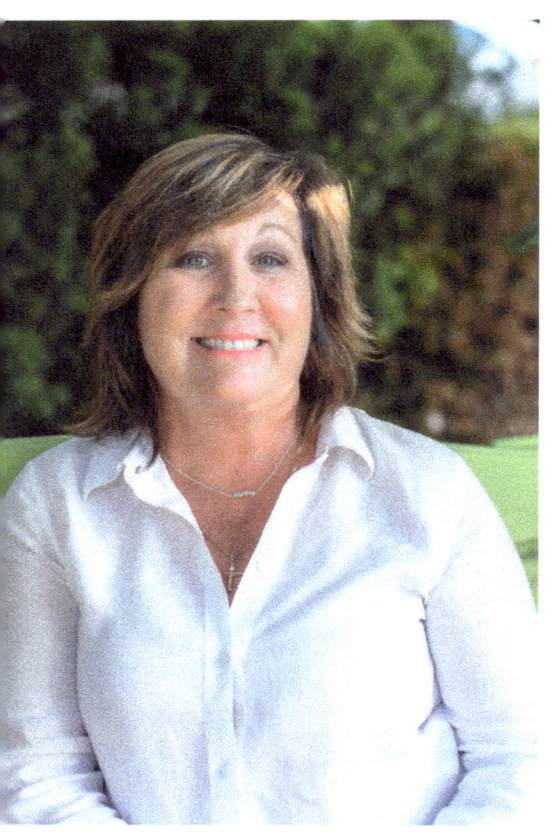

I'm thrilled to share what I can about my personal relationship with breast cancer. I say "relationship" because it's a constant in your life, for months or even years. In my diagnosis, I chose to be the stronger one in the relationship. It can and does hold a lot of power, but it's about how you manifest your power!

I'm very much a positive, outgoing, humorous woman. I did not (nor does anyone) expect to hear the diagnosis. Having been on the caregiving side with my husband as newlyweds, I learned very quickly never to ask "Why me?" or "Why he?" but rather "Why not?"

My path was to follow treatment, and I did not like it AT ALL—but

here I am! What I can say is this: Be sure to utilize kindness and gestures wherever you receive them! I took girlfriends wig shopping, and it was a hoot! I gained confidence wearing wigs that I never expected!

I remember the day I lost my eyelashes… Joan Lunden, a television host, shared that cancer had "erased" her face. At that point, I felt the same way—for a bit. Then I looked up breast cancer and eyelashes on the Internet. We are so fortunate to live in this era! I also chose hair loss as a chance to bring my sisters and friends together. They came over to sip wine and snip hair with me! Truly, it was the best idea!

So here I am, one year and a bit later! Period! I still love life and laughter, and I choose to live with—not die from—my relationship with breast cancer.

Also, prayer means everything to me, every single day!

All my love, friendship, and prayer. XOXO

By the way, breaking up with breast cancer… too much work!

Peggy Polewski

Wendy

June 17th, 2016, is a day I will never forget. Not only was it my brother's birthday, but it was also the day I was told the news that nobody wants to hear: *It looks like you have cancer.* It was a shock to me and my husband. My dad had a huge history of cancer on his side of the family, and my dad had passed away from cancer, but I did not expect to get diagnosed at the early age of 43. This was my biggest fear coming true. I had no history of breast cancer in my family on my mom's side or dad's side. At this moment, my body froze as well as my mind. My family physician's lips were moving, but my mind was stuck on the fact that I have cancer. My mind went to so many places: *I am going to die. I will not see my kids grow up. Is this really the end of my life?* My kids were too young to be without their mother. I couldn't sleep because I could not shut my mind off of all the terrible thoughts that ran through my

head. Luckily, my doctor prescribed medication to help me relax. I was always afraid to take medications like this, but I was so desperate to sleep and take my mind off of things. My first piece of advice: If your physician prescribes something like this, do not be afraid; this is something that may help you. But take them with caution.

The next step was my biopsy. I was still hoping for a benign tumor, but it was confirmed that, yes, I did indeed have cancer. I was diagnosed with Infiltrating Ductal Carcinoma, which was a common type of breast cancer. I was told that if there was any type of breast cancer to get, this was the one. Wow, I felt as if I had won the cancer lottery.

Next step was to be booked with the surgeon for a consult. This is where I felt comfort when the woman who answered the phone said that this wasn't a death sentence. I held on to those words, and still do to this day.

July 14th was my surgery date. This was another waiting game. I had to wait to make sure that the cancer had not spread to the lymph nodes and to find out the staging and the grade of the cancer. During this time, my husband and I took the kids away to our cottage in Michigan. Getting away was nice; it took my mind off of things for a little while. Then upon our return home, I had my follow up with the surgeon. My tumor was 5 cm, but luckily, had not affected my lymph nodes. My husband and I were both relieved.

It was at this point that I was referred to the cancer clinic; but before my consult, I was sent for a cat scan of the abdomen, a bone scan, and an ultrasound. More waiting! I always worried after every test, because my biggest fear was that the cancer would be somewhere else in my body—but the fact that it was not in the lymph nodes was a good indicator that it probably was contained. Everything came back clear, and I was booked for my consult with the oncologist at the end of August.

This was a scary moment for me, walking into that building. It made me think a lot about my dad and everything he had endured during

his cancer. And my mind also kept thinking, *I am too young for this. I don't belong here*! The oncologist recommended four rounds of chemotherapy, and then radiation. I was scared to death of chemo—you hear so many bad things, I didn't know what to expect. This is when I reached out to women and friends who had been through this before. This is one of the best things that I could have ever done. These women and my family were angels here on earth. I was finally ready to let people know I had breast cancer.

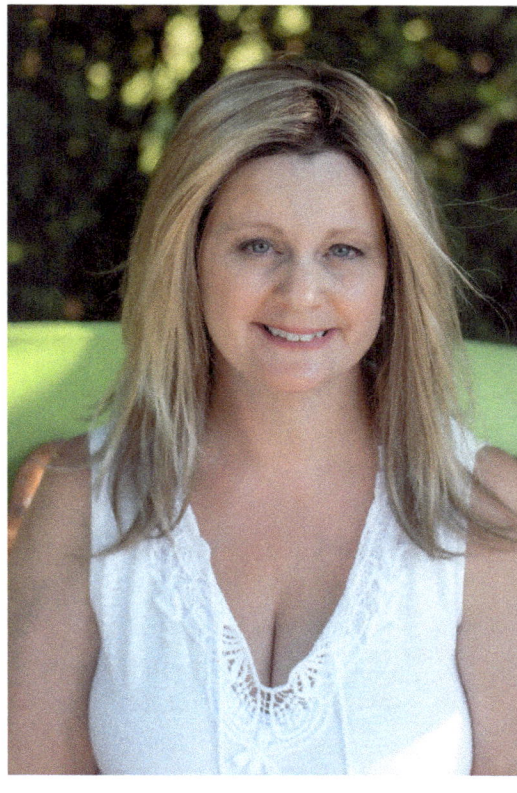

If there is another thing I can recommend to other women starting their journey, it would be to tell people what you are going through. Be angry, be upset, but don't be embarrassed to share with people, like I was. Don't be afraid to ask for help. Whether it be to watch the kids, cook you some meals, clean your house, give you gift certificates for restaurants—this helped me and my family a ton.

Another thing I can recommend is that if you are going to lose your hair, go shopping for wigs before it happens. This way, when you go to the wig salon they can recommend something close to your real hair. And bring a friend! Shopping for a wig was fun, and not as scary as I thought it would be—and Jackie made me feel great! After my first chemo treatment, my hair began falling out by strands. Every time I would gently pull my hair, pieces would blow away in the wind. It was the weirdest feeling. I felt as if this cancer was taking control—but then I took a bit of control back and cut my hair into a bob.

What I wasn't prepared for was when I washed my hair: It matted up into balls that I couldn't get out. This is when I felt my world came crumbling down. Nobody around me seemed to understand what this felt like, especially my husband. I know he tried, and I can't blame him for it. At this point, I reached out to one of my friends who was a hairdresser, and she gave me some really good advice. I could either let this cancer control me, or I could control this cancer. I wanted to shave my head, but I didn't have the nerve to do it. Instead I waited until the next day, and one of my other girlfriends gave me a beautiful pixie cut. Looking back, I should have just shaved it bald.

If you are going to lose your hair, just shave it bald. Take control of that cancer! Even after the pixie cut, the next morning I woke up to little pieces of hair on my pillow. My mother-in-law came over that day and shaved it for me. It actually felt good! It didn't look good at first—all I could think of was how I looked like my oldest brother! When you're used to long hair, it is hard to get used to something short. But just remember, it is hair, and it does grow back. In the end, what I came to realize was that it wasn't my hair that defined me—it was *me* that defines who I am.

When my first round of chemo came, I was nervous. How would this affect my body? Would I have a reaction? Luckily they give you medication to alleviate some of these symptoms. I think this helped me a lot. Being in the chemo suite was not at all what I expected. One thing I still felt was that I did not belong in there. There were people that appeared worse than myself—but what I did not expect were people who looked healthy like me. I was lucky to have my husband there, even just for company.

The day of chemotherapy, I felt great! I thought, *Wow! I could handle this, no problem!* But then, by the third day, it hit me; I was exhausted. I would wake up, get the kids a bowl of cereal, and even that took a lot out of me. I felt so bad that my kids and my husband had to see me like this. All I wanted to do was cry because I couldn't do what I would normally do. I had to be reassured by family and friends that this was

OK. I can't be Wonder Woman! My body needed rest. This is another thing I recommend: Rest a lot! Eat whatever you can, and try to drink lots of water to get those chemo toxins out of your body.

Three weeks after my chemo, I started my radiation. I had 20 treatments, which was every day for 5 weeks. I didn't notice any changes to my breasts until closer to the end of the treatment. My skin became very red, like a sunburn. I recommend getting a good moisturizer, and even if you don't notice any changes, continue using it because it will help in the end.

I am now a year cancer-free. And I still sometimes think, *Did that really happen?* Yes, it did. And it made me a stronger person. I now don't sweat the little or big things. I am a firm believer that everything happens for a reason. I now take time to appreciate all the things in life: my husband, my children, my mom, and all of my family and friends. If there is one thing that I have really learned, it's that life is short, but if you live it to the fullest, it can be the best shortest ride of your life. Enjoy every moment, even the ones that you don't expect. Stand up to cancer and show it who is boss!

Thank you to my husband, Mike, and to Jenna, Daniel, my mom, my mother- and father-in-law, my brothers and sisters, and all my other family and friends who helped me on this journey.

Wendy Probyn

Linda

My story began in 2014, when I was planning my son's wedding. I was feeling run down, and I thought it was because I'd been so busy, but decided to make an appointment with my family doctor.

My doctor did a complete physical, as it had been two years since my last one. A couple of weeks later, they called to let me know they had seen something on my mammogram. I returned for a biopsy, and three

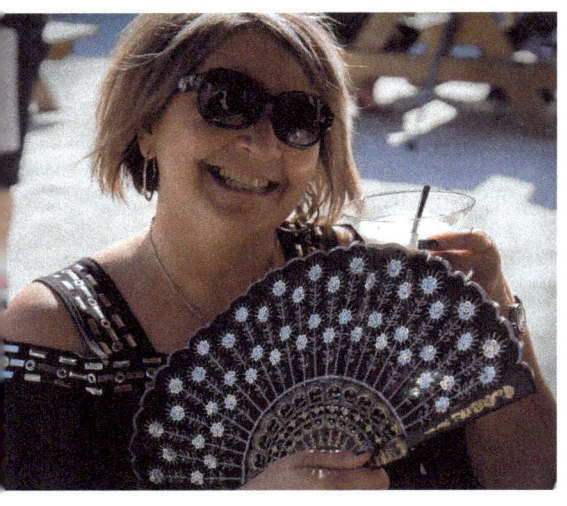

weeks after my son's wedding, I was diagnosed with stage 3 ductal carcinoma breast cancer.

I was devastated and went through many different emotions. But my family and friends were amazing and never let me get down.

I was diagnosed on November 4th and had a double mastectomy less than three weeks later. My surgeon, Dr. Shael Liebman, was wonderful and caring. He took very good care of me and my family. He was attentive and made everyone feel at ease. In January of 2015, I began nine months of chemo, and then six weeks of radiation. It was tough, with good and bad days. I always had family and friends with me when I needed, and if I wanted to be alone, they understood.

The strength I found was something I never knew I had. But I find that cancer patients dig deep and find that strength to continue the fight, to be positive for themselves and, yes, also for their family and friends. I continued to keep life as normal as possible. And I always said, "Let me try and do it first; if I can't do it, then help me please." I always say that a strong person will fall, but will always get up, cry, and move on. And if it hurts, keep going.

Always be thankful for what you have and know that you are loved.

Tell yourself, no matter hard it is or how hard it gets, *I'M GOING TO MAKE IT.*

Linda Santos

Cathy

I was diagnosed with stage 3 breast cancer on March 12, 2015. Wow, I was all by myself. But I'm doing good now. Without having lived through "those days," I wouldn't be as strong or as peaceful as I am today.

I did not realize what was in store for me. Being a healthy and knowledgeable person, I decided on an integrative approach to my health plan. I've nothing against the standard chemo/radiation therapy, but I believe in healthy living via juices—no dairy, no red meat, no sugar, no white or refined anything.

I welcome women to contact me and consult my Facebook pages that feature juices. It has been the hardest year of my life—but I know we can do it, ladies!

Cathy Sebben

Rachel

The words spoken by my 8-year-old daughter Olivia are words that I'll never forget: "Mom, you don't *look* like you have cancer. Do you *feel* like you have it?" To be honest, I couldn't tell I had cancer, and I didn't look like a cancer patient either. YET. Funny thing is, cancer isn't what makes us look sick—the treatments are. I didn't start to look sick until I was well into my chemo treatments. The loss of hair and lifelessness in your face, that's from the chemo, and it builds up over time.

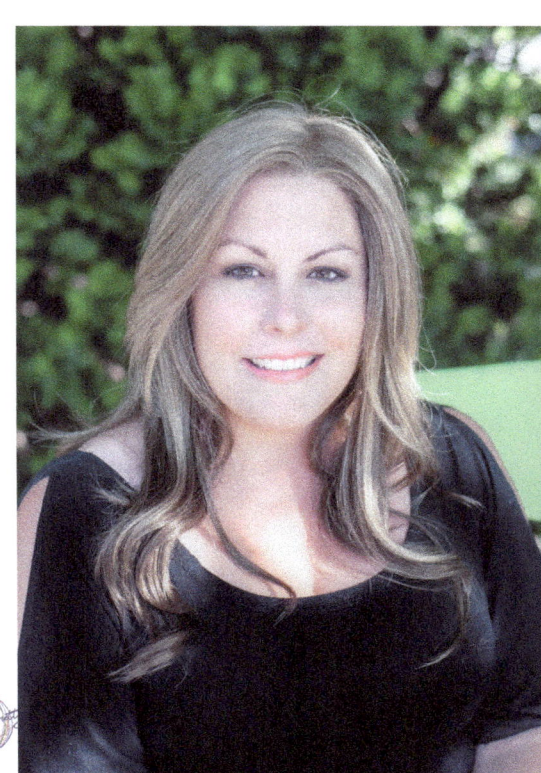

I learned that doing things to make you feel good is what keeps you strong. My advice: Get a wig or wear a fancy head covering. Put your make-up on, even though half of your eyelashes are missing. Take a shower, get dressed. And go to the Look Good Feel Better program at the hospital for free products and awesome advice. I had no idea that I wasn't supposed to be using anti-aging products while undergoing chemo. It was burning my eyelids, and I was unaware that I was doing it to myself.

And LAUGH! It really is the best medicine. I rely on my friends for some good therapy through laughter. I most recently bought a Jeep because I said it's the only way I'll look good with my top off now! My husband, Mike, who has been my rock in all of this, will often shake his head at me and my ridiculous humor—but he knows that's what I need to cope. He always made me smile every day, no matter how sick I became.

Radiation builds up over time, and although everyone is different, you will probably burn and be very uncomfortable. They provide creams for open sores, and my sister-in-law got me a giant aloe plant to help soothe the unopened wounds. Radiation will also exhaust you—so SLEEP! Your body needs it to heal and recover from all the poison that has been put into it.

My cancer was very uncooperative; the chemo didn't seem to work and my tumors continued to grow throughout treatment. We had to stop and do a bilateral mastectomy, so I got a little break from chemo. It was very emotional to lose the "girls"; they were a very big part of what made me a woman. My hair, lashes, eyebrows, and breasts were all stripped away from me, and I gained a good 30 pounds from the steroids they put me on. I'd look in the mirror and wonder where that beautiful woman I once knew had gone to.

I REALLY struggled, and it wasn't easy. But the good news is: I'M ALIVE! And I'll be here to see my children graduate and get married. I'm here to grow old with my husband. My hair is starting to grow back, and my lashes and brows are beautiful again! I still have some

weight to lose, and unfortunately I can't grow my breasts back, but I feel womanly again! I'm currently deciding on whether breast reconstruction is right for me. I know many women get reconstruction done, but some choose to embrace their new flat chest or choose to wear breast prostheses. While I decide, I choose mostly the flat route—but occasionally the "new girls" come out, and it's great to have the option! My sons, who are very wise for their young ages of 15 and 11, told me that I look great the way I am, and they'd rather I didn't undergo another surgery after all I have been through; it brought tears to my eyes!

Breast cancer is scary. It's not a pink candle in your inbox with the words: "Keep this going to fight cancer." It's not a post on your timeline that reads "Banana" to help spread awareness and keep the men guessing. Breast cancer is CTs, X-rays, MRIs, bone scans, biopsies, surgeries, amputations, scars, radiation, chemo, IVs, blood tests, multiple medications, injections, and numerous appointments. It's fear, worry, hate, anger, confusion, sadness, loneliness, hopelessness, anxiety, pain, nausea, vomiting, and having the Cancer Centre phone number in your address book under "favorites." This is all normal, and your feelings will be like a rollercoaster ride of emotions.

This was my reality—but it was only a bump in my road, and one day, *you*'ll be writing your story about being a *survivor*, like me!

You got this!

Rachel Spadotto

Susan

I encourage all of those facing a serious diagnosis to be proactive, research, educate yourself, and to question doctors. It's your life. It's your body.

Of course, take care of yourself: Stick to clean, healthy eating, and exercise whenever you are able to—walking is especially beneficial to the mind and body.

Pamper yourself. Epsom salt soaks flush toxins and relax muscles. Use wonderful healing scents. I used St. Francis Farms Calendula salve on my skin before radiation and on top of prescribed medical creams during and after the treatments. It stains, so wear a T-shirt or use a bed pad, but it keeps the area supple and helps it to heal. I had open areas that healed nicely as a result.

I also selected a card for myself for inspiration. It had a beautiful image on the front with the words, "May you have patience with all things… Above all, may you have patience with yourself." It sits on my dresser. It's a little thing that has brought me comfort and reminded me not to be so hard on myself. So many things can inspire: nature, looking at the sky against tree branches, spirituality, embracing forces all around us to strengthen and heal. My Reiki healer has been a gift. Crystals also emanate powerful healing energy. Journaling has provided not only a record of my journey to healing, but also an outlet to express my emotions and aspirations.

Gratitude is something I've experienced continually, for the people who have shown kindness and generosity, and for nature, books, films, and programs or words that meant so much. It's so beneficial to share and encourage others going through the same process.

I would say to all: DON'T JUST SURVIVE—THRIVE! At the end of this journey, you'll truly be reborn. Find your tribe. Create. Grow a garden. Make art. Write. Travel. Embrace life; don't hide from it.

BE GLORIOUSLY FIERCE & LOVING! SHINE! SPARKLE! ILLUMINATE!

Thank you for this opportunity to share.

Gratefully,

Susan Szucs

Jen

It's terrifying to hear those dreaded words: *You have cancer.* At 30 years old, I did not think I'd have to worry about buying bras with inserts that would make me look "normal" or about which wig would look most natural on me.

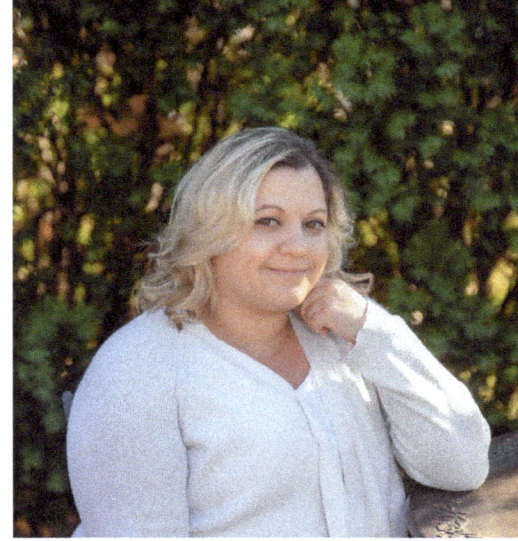

My diagnosis came after being told I have the BRCA mutation, which led me to a routine mammogram. I had no symptoms. I felt great. I was the healthiest I had ever been. How did I have breast cancer?

I did everything I could to make sure I did not lose myself during this time. I had a double mastectomy with immediate reconstruction. I shaved my head before chemo had the chance to take my hair from me. I was not letting this disease take me the way it took my father, grandmother, and countless other people. *I* was in control, not the cancer.

I bought different styles of wigs—long, short, curly, straight, brown, blonde, red—you name it, I had it. If this was my new "norm," why not have fun with it? I rarely left my house without wearing one of my wigs. I'd even wear them to chemo treatments. They made me feel beautiful. They made me feel like my old self.

I played around a lot with make-up—different colored eye shadows and bold lipsticks. YouTube tutorials became my go-to for ideas. Some days I felt like a little kid playing in my mom's make-up bag.

I kept as active as my body would allow. On my good days, I went for walks or did yoga. I took probiotics and milk thistle. I drank dandelion and ginger tea. On days I could not eat as much, I'd always have an iced capp.

I joined online forums for women who had breast cancer. Some were recently diagnosed, some were going through treatment, and some were survivors. It was nice to have people to talk to who knew how I was feeling. We shared tips and tricks on what worked for us.

Everyone will give their opinions about what you should do. But the truth is, you'll find what works for you. Maybe it's a wig that makes you feel good about yourself, or a new pair of shoes. Maybe it's a brand-new red lipstick.

Just know, whether you are having a good or a bad day, you are tougher than you think. You are beautiful inside and out. You are a fighter!

Jen Teti

Jane

Reaching out for help is important. Many people don't know what to do or say to you. Let them know what you need. There are services at the Cancer Centre like dieticians, social workers, and volunteers. Utilize these. It only takes a phone call, and it's free. I read morning devotions from *Power Thoughts* by Joyce Meyer. It's a great way to start my day.

Jane McGinnis

Lisa

I was 30 years old, a young mom, and a new bride when I was diagnosed with cancer! My world was turned upside-down the day the doctor told me. I was overcome by fear and sadness, not to mention a will to win.

The thing that probably helped me most while I was going through this was my amazing husband, who promised me daily that I was going to be okay. I also surrounded myself with friends who kept me busy by taking me to chemo, the garden center, out for coffee, everything

that ladies do with each other. My family, including brothers, sister-in-law, and parents, were also a tremendous support. My daughter was seven at the time, and my desire to travel with her also played a big role in my healing. I took her to Disney World in the middle of my treatment, PICC line in my bicep and all!

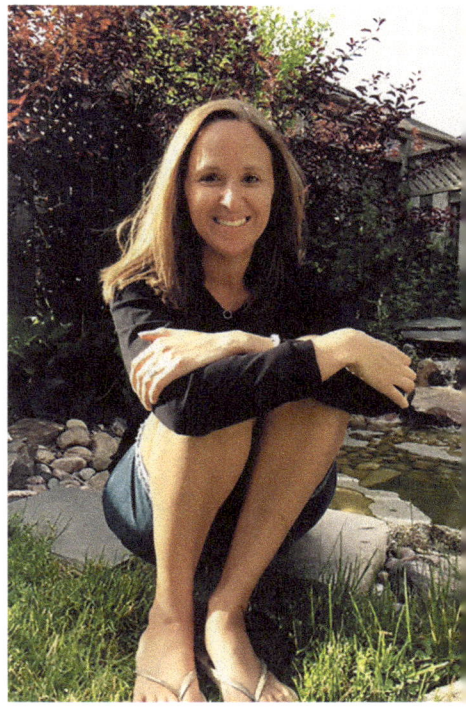

Another thing that made my journey bearable was my therapist. She was essential in helping me pick up the pieces. During one session, she gave me a bookmark featuring the Serenity Prayer. I'm not a regular at church; however, anytime I was feeling dark, I'd recite this verse:

God, grant me the serenity to accept the things I can't change, the courage to change the things I can, and the wisdom to know the difference.

Today, I'm proud to say that I'm helping patients with their journey through my company, Aya Covers, which provides PICC line covers to patients. It really is the little things that make a difference!

Thank you!

Lisa Thompson

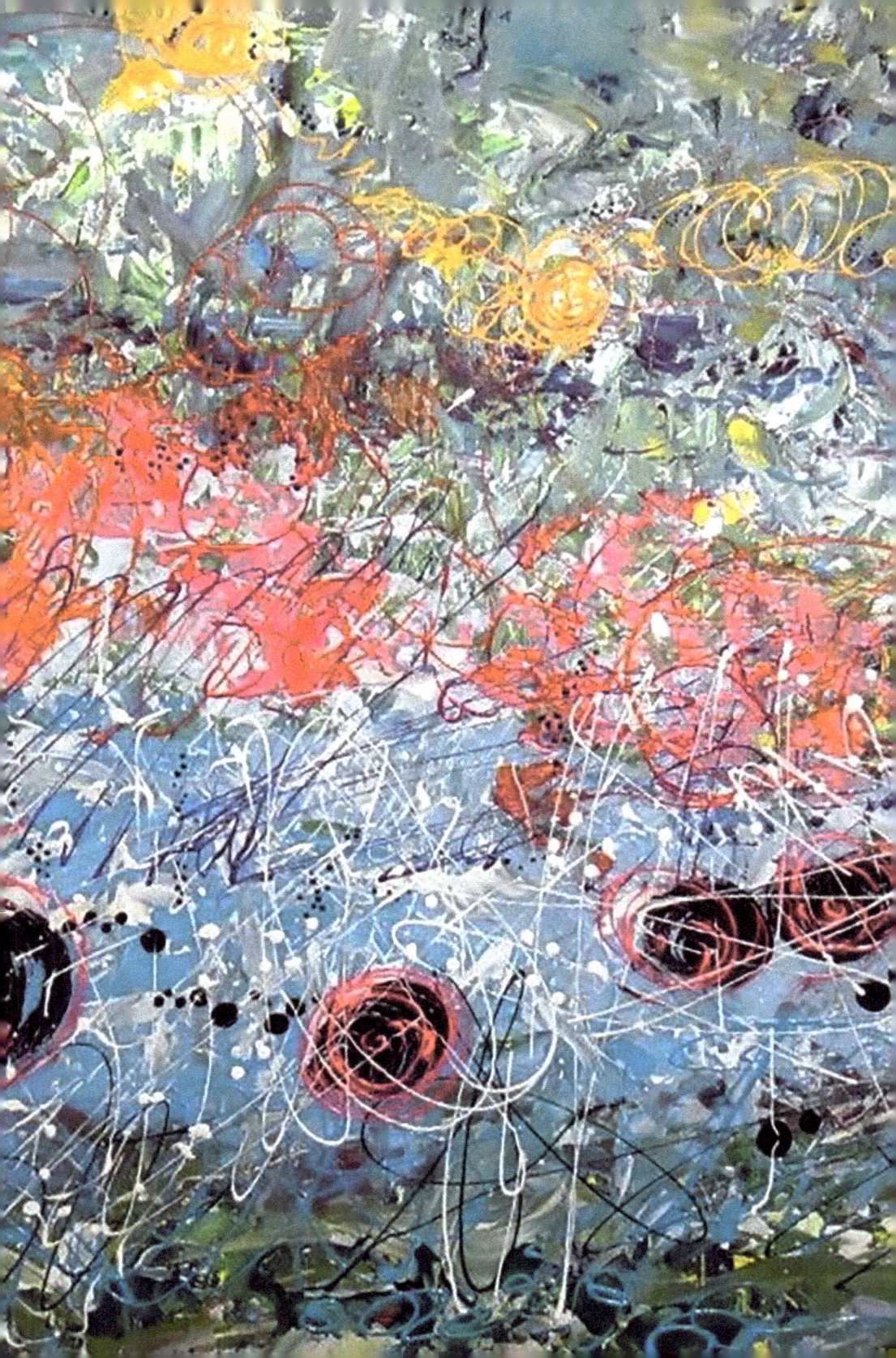

"Everything will be okay in the end; if it's not okay, it's not the end." Ever since I was diagnosed with breast cancer, this quote has been my mantra. These words have been my anthem, my inspiration, my comfort, and my prayer."

—Giuliana Rancic, author, fashion and beauty expert, television personality, breast cancer survivor

. . . .

12
Closing Thoughts

I wish each one of you a full recovery with the best possible treatment and manageable side effects. My hope for you, as you move toward recovery, is that you feel a weight lifted and take comfort in knowing that you can be confident, maintain your dignity, and feel beautiful every step of the way.

It's an honor for me to be able to help women like you, daily. I wish I could meet every single one of you. Please know you're in my heart. We are all connected, and I can promise you that positive energy is coming your way. I believe we are put on this earth to help one another. And I know that, one day, you'll be fortunate enough to get the opportunity to pay it forward, as I have.

Here's to you and to healing pretty!

Brightest Blessings,

Jackie Apostol-Pizzuti

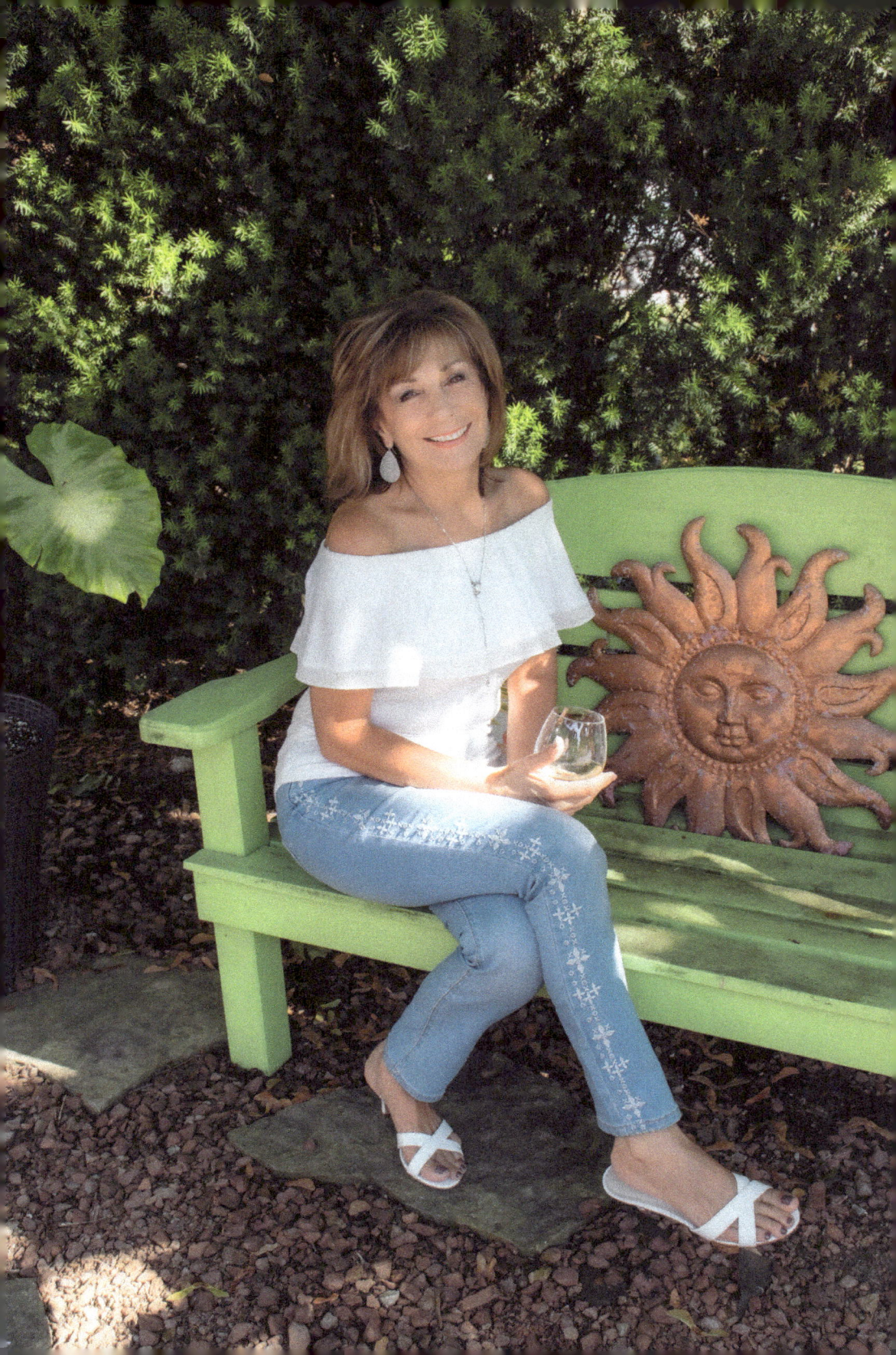

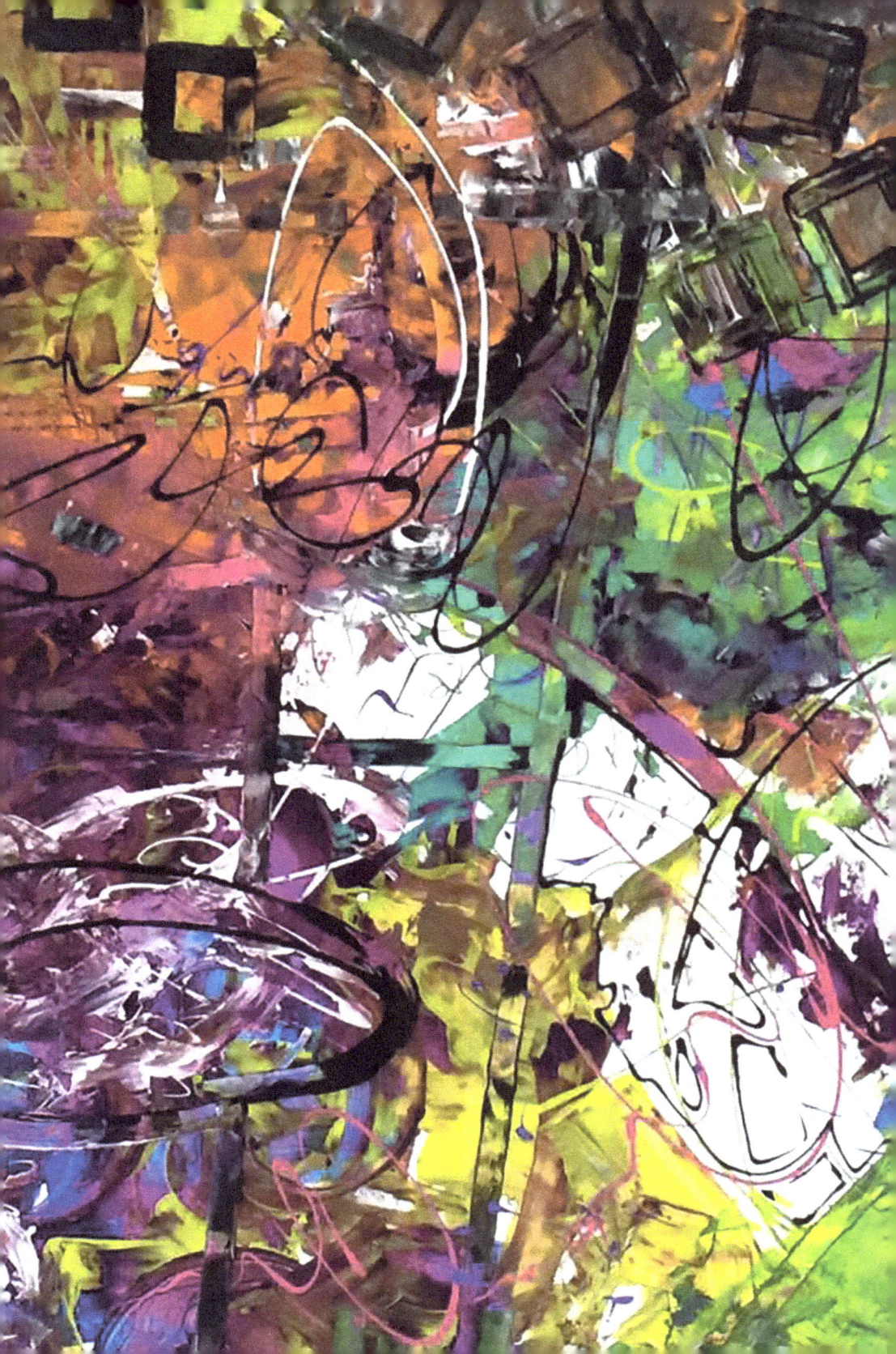

"My cancer scare changed my life. I'm grateful for every new healthy day I have. It has helped me prioritize my life."

—Olivia Newton-John, singer-songwriter, actress, entrepreneur, activist, author, breast cancer survivor

Appendix A

A handy checklist list for all your
cancer self-care essentials

Whether you're shopping for yourself or a loved one, I believe this list may be helpful.

After a friend of mine finished reading *Healing Pretty* (when it was still just a manuscript), she was inspired to put together a lovely and thoughtful gift for her best friend who was recently diagnosed with cancer. She made a list of the products mentioned in the book, went shopping, and put together a gift basket filled with everything she thought would be helpful.

To make things easier, I've created a convenient list of items I've handpicked from *Healing Pretty* that should be easy to find at your local drugstore or cancer care boutique. I've also included some other helpful items and ideas.

Skincare

Aveeno Soothing
   Bath Treatments.
Aveeno Skin Relief
   Soothing Shampoo

Aveeno Intense Relief
   Hand Cream
Clinique Redness
   Solutions Makeup

Garnier Ombrelle Complete
      Lotion SPF 30
Ivory Liquid Body Soap
Neutrogena Facial Moisturizer

Vichy Aqualia Thermal
      Eye Roll-On
Virgin Coconut Oil
Vitamin E Cream

Mouth and Lips

Biotène Toothpaste
Biotène Moisturizing
      Mouth Wash
Blistex Lip Medex

SalivaSure Lozenges
Lemon candies
Ginger candy/chews

Garments and Accessories

PICC line cover
Seat belt cushion
Underarm breast pillow

Seasonal hats
Pre-tied head scarves
Sleep cap

Chemo Days

Journal book
Comfy blanket
Fuzzy socks
Warm scarf
Shawl
A good book (*Healing Pretty!*)
Skin lotion
Hand sanitizer
Words of encouragement,
      inspirational quotes
Magazine
Coloring book, crayons
Crossword/Sudoku
Board games
Deck of cards

Sleeping mask
Something from home that
      brings you comfort
      (stuffed animal, etc.)
Tote bag
Music

Other Ways to Help Someone Going Through Treatment

Gift Certificates

- Restaurants (take-out is always appreciated)
- Local companies who plan and deliver meals
- Cancer care boutiques

Personal Promise Cards. You can get creative with this. Here are just a few ideas to help get you going:

- Home-cooked meal delivered
- House cleaning/outdoor maintenance
- Babysitting/pet sitting
- General errands
- Picking up prescriptions
- Groceries
- Driving

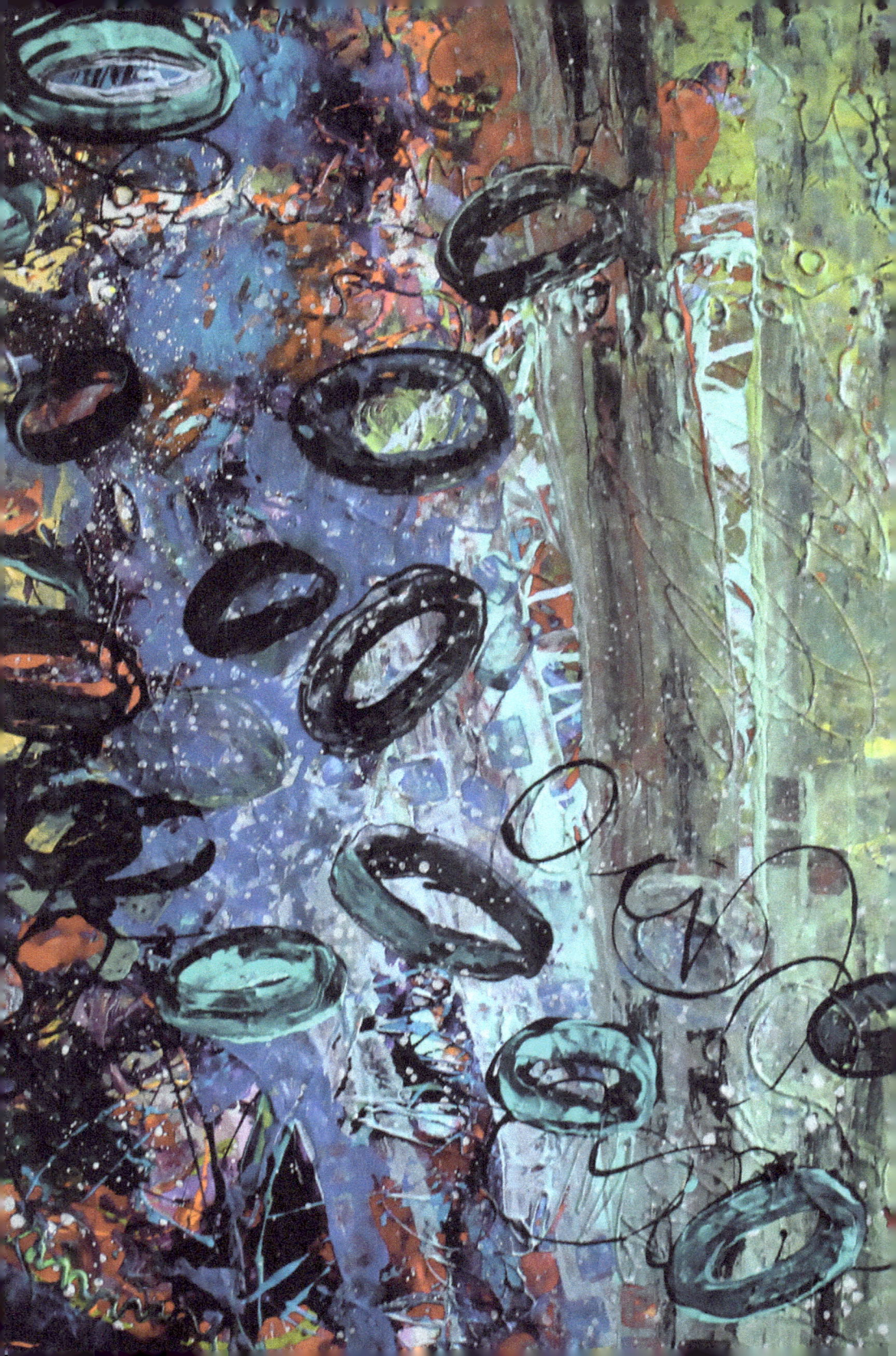

. . . .

Appendix B

Healing resources

Here's a handy reference of the products and services mentioned in *Healing Pretty*, plus a few more.

This list will change and expand as I discover new items. Please check www.healingprettybook.com for updates. There, I also welcome you to share your great finds!

Garments and Accessories

Aya Covers: PICC Line Covers
www.ayacovers.com

Chemo Beanies
www.chemobeanies.com

Coolibar: Sun Protective Clothing
www.coolibar.com

Cool-jams: Moisture-Wicking Sleepwear and Bedding
www.cool-jams.com

CS: Ostomy Pouch Covers
www.cspouchcovers.com

Grandma's Hands: Ostomy and Urostomy Covers
www.grandmashands.ca

HAPARI: Mastectomy-Friendly Swimwear
www.hapari.com

Haralee: Moisture-wicking Sleepwear and Bedding
www.haralee.com

HysterSisters: Woman-to-Woman Hysterectomy Support
www.hystersisters.com

Juzo: Compression Sleeves and Stockings
www.juzousa.com

LympheDIVAs: Fashionable Compression Sleeves
www.lymphedivas.com

Na' Scent: Ostomy Odor Control
www.nascent4u.com

Ostomy Secrets: Panties, Wraps, and Swimwear
www.ostomysecrets.com

Pink Lotus: Billow Heart Breast Pillow
www.pinklotus.com

Pink Pepper Co: Mastectomy Chest Pillow with a Shield, U Supports, and Wings
www.pinkpepperco.com

Post Op Panty: Post-Operative Compression Panties
www.postoppanty.com

Radiant Wrap: Fashionable Clothing During Radiation Treatment
www.theradiantwrap.com

Reboundwear: Post-Surgical Tops, Jackets, Pants, and Hospital Gowns, endorsed by medical professionals
www.reboundwear.com

Sleek Sleeves: PICC Line Covers
www.sleeksleeves.com

Stealth Belt: Ostomy Wraps and Belts
www.stealthbelt.com

The Brobe: Post Recovery Attire
www.thebrobe.com

Vegan Ostomy: Tips, Care, and Resources
www.veganostomy.ca

Wigs to Wellness & The Mastectomy Boutique: Seat Belt Cushions
www.wigstowellness.com

Skincare

Dermaflage: Scar and Wrinkle Filler, Scar Removal Cream
www.dermaflage.com

Jean's Cream: Radiation Burns
www.jeanscream.com

Lindi Skin: Chemo and Radiation Skincare
www.lindiskin.com

Mederma: Scar Cream
www.mederma.ca

Ocean Bottom Soap Company: Organic and Chemical-Free Products
www.oceanbottomsoap.com

Scar Away: Sheets & Gels
www.myscaraway.com

Soap Chef: Organic and Chemical-Free Products
www.soapchefmadetoorder.ca

Make-Up

BeautyCounter: Non-Toxic, Chemical-Free Cosmetics
www.beautycounter.com

GrandeLASH-MD: Eyelash Growth Serum
www.grandecosmetics.com

LashyBrows: Eyebrow Wigs
www.lashybrows.com

Latisse: Eyelash Growth Serum
www.latisse.com

Look Good Feel Better Program: Beauty Techniques
www.lookgoodfeelbetter.org

NaturaLash: Eyebrow Wigs
www.naturalash.com

Rapid Brow: Eyebrow Enhancing Serum
www.rapidlash.com/products/rapidbrow

RMS Beauty: Non-Toxic, Chemical Free Cosmetics
www.rmsbeauty.com

SurvivorEyes: Brow Styling Kits
www.survivoreyes.com

Mastectomy Products

American Breast Care: Breast Prostheses, Bras, and Post Mastectomy
Healing Kits
www.americanbreastcare.com

Nordstrom: Breast Prosthesis Program
www.nordstrom.com

Pink Perfect: Custom-Made Prosthetic Nipples
www.pink-perfect.com

Prairie Wear: Post-Surgical Bras & Binders
www.prairie.world

Wigs to Wellness & The Mastectomy Boutique: Breast Pillows
www.wigstowellness.com

Other Resources

Canadian Lymphedema Framework: List of Provincial
Lymphedema Associations
www.canadalymph.ca

CancerCare: Free Counseling, Education, Support Services, &
Resources In-Person and Online (US)
www.cancercare.org

Environmental Working Group (EWG): Databases of
Beauty, Personal Care and Cleaning Products Ingredients and
Toxicity Ratings
www.ewg.org/skindeep

National Lymphedema Network: Information and Resources (US)
www.lymphnet.org

Yoga4Cancer: Free Research-Based Yoga
www.y4c.com

Other Side Effects

Biotene: Dry Mouth, Mouth Sores, Oral Thrush
www.biotene.ca

Penguin Cold Caps: Hair Loss from Chemo
www.penguincoldcaps.com

Sea-band: Nausea
www.sea-band.com

Térapo Médik Well Being Care Kit: Hair and Scalp Care During and
After Treatment
www.terapomedik.com

Sexuality and Cancer

American Association of Sex Educators, Counselors, and Therapists
(AASECT): Sex Therapists
www.aasect.org

American Cancer Society: *Sex and The Woman With Cancer*
www.cancer.org

Anne Katz, Dr.: Sex Expert for People with Cancer
www.drannekatz.com

Astroglide: Vaginal Lubricant
www.astroglide.com

K-Y SILKE-E: Vaginal Moisturizer
www.k-y.ca

Livestrong: "Female Sexual Health After Cancer"
www.livestrong.org

National Association of Social Workers (NASW): Sex Therapists
www.helpstartshere.org

National Cancer Institute: Self Image and Sexuality
www.cancer.gov

Replens Silky Smooth: Vaginal Moisturizer
www.replens.com

Stupid Cancer: Young Adult Cancer Advocacy, Research, and Support
www.stupidcancer.org

YES – The Organic Intimacy Company: Plant-Based Vaginal Moisturizers and Lubricants
www.yesyesyes.org

Wigs and Headwear

Artizara: Hijabs/ Islam Headwear
www.artizara.com

Envy Wigs: Envy and Sherri Shepard Wigs
www.envywigs.com

Fortune Wigs: Kosher Wigs
www.fortunewigs.com

Headline It: No Sweat Wig Liners
www.headlineit.com

Jon Renau: Wigs and Headwear
www.jonrenau.com

The Wig Fix: Gripper Band
www.therenatural.com

Tichel Volumizer: Pre-Padded Cap
www.etsy.com/ca/market/tichel_volumizer

Truly You Hair Solution Centre: Custom Made Wigs
www.trulyyou.ca

Vivica Fox: Wigs
www.vivicafox.com

Wrapunzel: Tichels/Jewish Headwear
www.wrapunzel.com

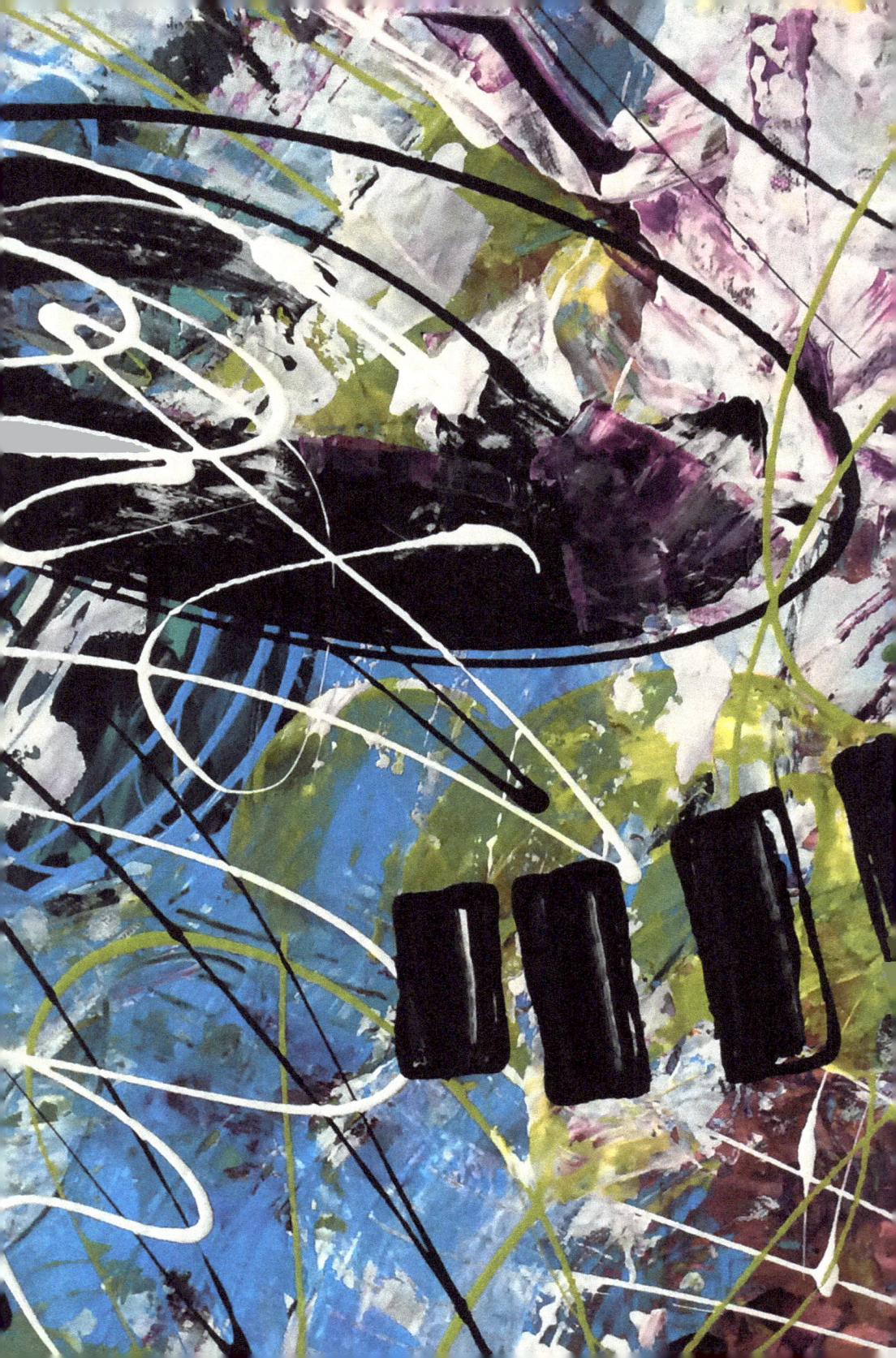

Additional Acknowledgements

Here's to our Soul-ebrity Sisters!

They are strong and courageous, just like you. They lived with cancer and fought to survive, just like you. They had chemo, radiation, and surgeries, just like you. They endured adverse side effects, they cried and feared, just like you. They made the best of a bad situation, just like you. We are all the same—cancer has no boundaries. Fame, power, money, color, gender, race, religion—it doesn't matter, no one is protected, and no one has the power to make it go away. In this unbalanced world, cancer is the equalizer; it makes us humble, and cognitive of the fact that we are all one, we are all sisters.

Good Morning America's Robin Roberts quotes her mother: "Make your mess your message."

That's what our Soul-ebrity Sisters have done. They give to us a very special gift: their voices. They've openly shared their experiences and have brought about public awareness of this dreadful disease. They're our advocate and our hope; they're our voice. They've inspired, empowered, enlightened, and educated us. They are actively and passionately involved in charities, foundations, and causes. They're all incredible women who shine. They're warriors.

Their wisdom has been sprinkled throughout *Healing Pretty*. I hope you've been uplifted by their words of encouragement.

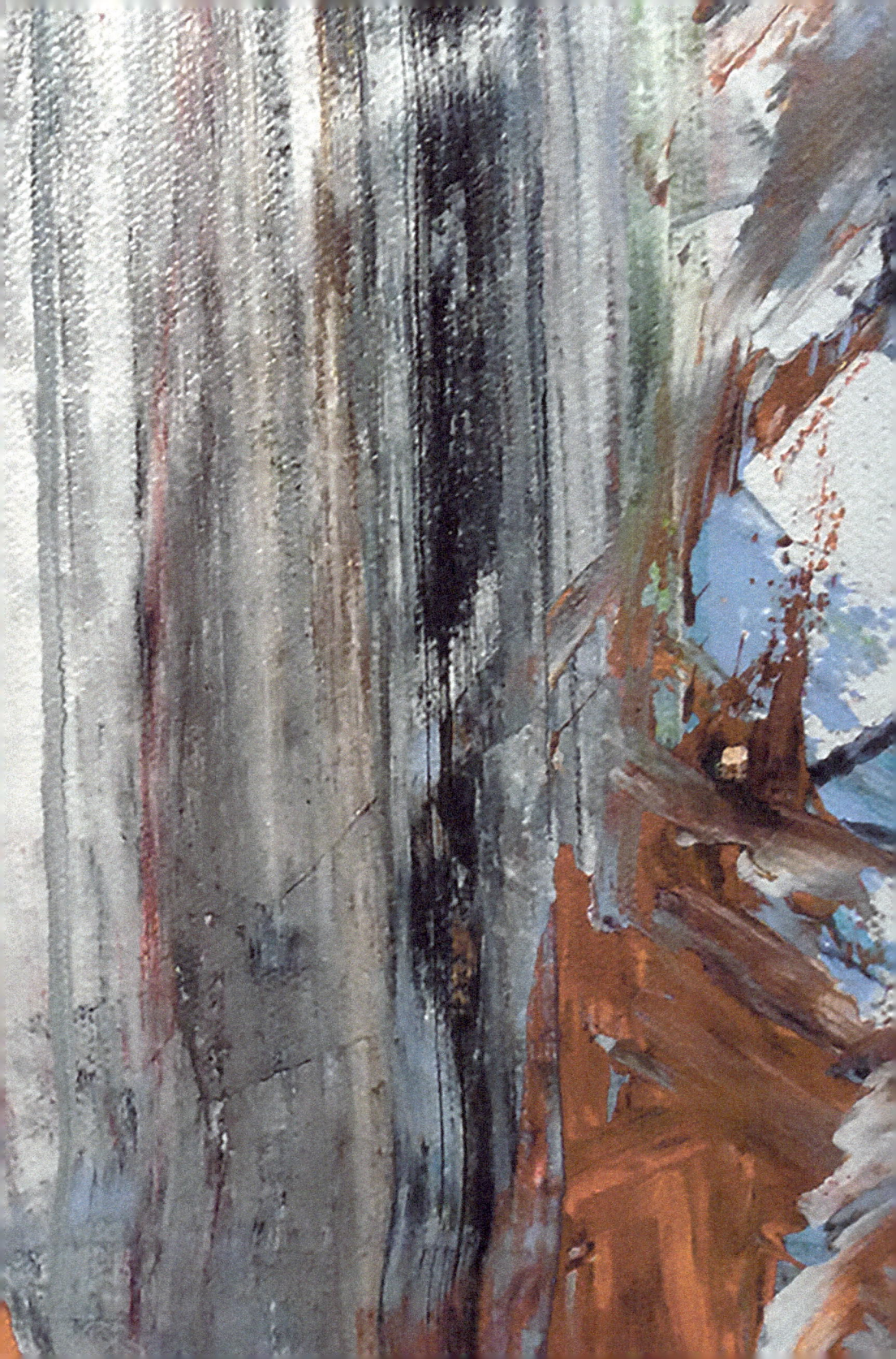

References

Alkon, Cheryl. "Tips for Tackling Chemo Brain." Everyday Health. com. https://www.everydayhealth.com/breast-cancer/symptoms/tips-tackling-chemo-brain/ (accessed May 16, 2019).

American Cancer Society. "Breast Reconstruction Options." Cancer. org. http://www.cancer.org/cancer/breastcancer/moreinformation/breastreconstructionaftermastectomy/breast-reconstruction-after-mastectomy-br-recon-choices (accessed August 26, 2016).

American Cancer Society. "Cancer, Sex, and the Female Body." Cancer.org. http://www.cancer.org/treatment/treatmentsandsideeffects/physicalsideeffects/sexualsideeffectsinwomen/sexualityforthewoman/sexuality-for-women-with-cancer-cancer-sex-sexuality (accessed September 8, 2016).

American Cancer Society. "For People at Risk of Lymphedema." Cancer.org. https://www.cancer.org/treatment/treatments-and-side-effects/physical-side-effects/lymphedema/for-people-at-risk-of-lymphedema.html (accessed August 24, 2016).

American Cancer Society. "Life after Cancer." Cancer.org. https://www.cancer.org/treatment/survivorship-during-and-after-treatment/be-healthy-after-treatment/life-after-cancer.html (accessed September 19, 2017).

American Cancer Society. "Lymphedema: What Every Woman with Breast Cancer Should Know." Cancer.org. http://www.cancer.org/treatment/treatmentsandsideeffects/physicalsideeffects/lymphedema/

whateverywomanwithbreastcancershouldknow/index (accessed
August 24, 2016).

American Cancer Society. "Physical Activity and the Cancer Patient."
Cancer.org. http://www.cancer.org/treatment/survivorshipduringan-
daftertreatment/stayingactive/physical-activity-and-the-cancer-patient
(accessed September 25, 2016).

American Cancer Society. "Treating Sexual Problems for Women with
Cancer." Cancer.org. https://www.cancer.org/treatment/treatments-
and-side-effects/physical-side-effects/fertility-and-sexual-side-effects/
sexuality-for-women-with-cancer/problems.html (accessed May
11, 2019).

American Cancer Society. "Treatments and Side Effects." Cancer.org.
https://www.cancer.org/treatment/treatments-and-side-effects.html
(accessed May 8, 2016).

American Cancer Society. "What to Expect after Breast
Reconstruction Surgery." Cancer.org. http://www.cancer.org/cancer/
breastcancer/moreinformation/breastreconstructionaftermastectomy/
breast-reconstruction-after-mastectomy-after-surgery (accessed
September 1, 2016).

American Dental Association. "Cancer: Taking Care of Your Teeth
after Treatment." Mouth Healthy. https://www.mouthhealthy.org/en/
az-topics/c/cancer-after-treatment (accessed May 11, 2019).

American Society of Clinical Oncology. "Side Effects of Radiation
Therapy." Cancer.net. https://www.cancer.net/navigating-cancer-care/
how-cancer-treated/radiation-therapy/side-effects-radiation-therapy
(accessed January 19, 2017).

Banker, Angela. "Chemo Brain Is Real And Here Are 10 Symptoms
Associated With It." TheBreastCancerSite.com. https://blog.thebreast-
cancersite.greatergood.com/angela-chemo-brain-list/ (accessed August
6, 2019).

Beauty & Hair. "The Differences between Human Hair and Synthetic Hair Wigs." Wigs.com. https://www.wigs.com/pages/the-differences-between-human-hair-synthetic-hair (accessed July 1, 2017).

Brain & Spine Foundation. "Craniotomy." Brainandspine.org. http://www.brainandspine.org.uk/our-publications/our-fact-sheets/craniotomy/ (accessed May 2, 2017).

Breastcancer.org. "Before You Begin Chemotherapy." Breastcancer.org. http://www.breastcancer.org/treatment/chemotherapy/process/before (accessed July 1, 2017).

Breastcancer.org. "Cold Caps and Scalp Cooling Systems." Breastcancer.org. https://www.breastcancer.org/tips/hair_skin_nails/cold-caps (accessed August 26, 2016).

Breastcancer.org. "Compression Sleeves and Garments." Breastcancer.org. http://www.breastcancer.org/treatment/lymphedema/treatments/sleeves (accessed August, 2016).

Breastcancer.org. "Reducing Lymphedema and Flare-Up Risk: Things to Do." Breastcancer.org. https://www.breastcancer.org/treatment/lymphedema/reduce_risk/do (accessed September 14, 2019).

Breastcancer.org. "Routinely Removing Axillary Lymph Nodes May Not Make Sense for Many Women." Breastcancer.org. https://www.breastcancer.org/research-news/20110208 (accessed September 14, 2019).

BreastReconstruction.org Medical Board. "Nipple Areola Tattoo." Breastreconstruction.org. http://www.breastreconstruction.org/SecondaryProcedures/NippleAreolaTattoo.html (accessed February 26, 2019).

British Acupuncture Council. "Can Acupuncture Help with Scar Tissue?" Acupuncture.org.uk. https://www.acupuncture.org.uk/public-content/public-ask-an-expert/ask-an-expert-body/

ask-an-expert-body-skin-conditions/can-acupuncture-help-with-scar-tissue.html (accessed May 10, 2018).

Brown, Mackenzie, and Jennifer Graham Kizer. "Edie Falco Talks about Her Breast Cancer Journey." Health.com. https://www.health.com/health/article/0,,20411264,00.html (accessed December 14, 2016).

Buttimer, Angela, and Dennis Buttimer. "Cancer Care and the 4 C's of Mindfulness." *Huffington Post.* http://www.huffingtonpost.com/entry/cancer-care-and-the-4-cs-of-mindfulness_us_57f79a82e4b0b665ad817d3d (accessed September 19, 2017).

Cafasso, Jacquelyn. "Treatment for Hypertrophic Scars." Healthline.com.https://www.healthline.com/health/hypertrophic-scar-treatment (accessed May 13, 2018).

Canadian Cancer Society. "Infection." Cancer.ca. http://www.cancer.ca/en/cancer-information/diagnosis-and-treatment/managing-side-effects/infection/?region=on (accessed May 2, 2017).

Canadian Cancer Society. "Sexuality and Cancer." Cancer.ca. http://www.cancer.ca/en/cancer-information/cancer-journey/living-with-cancer/sexuality-and-cancer/?region=bc (accessed September 8, 2016).

Cancer.net Editorial Board. "Hair Loss or Alopecia." Cancer.net. http://www.cancer.net/navigating-cancer-care/side-effects/hair-loss-or-alopecia (accessed January 3, 2017).

Cancer.Net. "Fertility Concerns and Preservation for Women." Cancer.net. https://www.cancer.net/navigating-cancer-care/dating-sex-and-reproduction/fertility-concerns-and-preservation-women (accessed September 12, 2019).

Cerner Multum Inc. "Votrient." Drugs.com. https://www.drugs.com/votrient.html (accessed September 5, 2017).

Chen, Joyce. "Giuliana Rancic Celebrates Being Five Years Cancer-Free." *Us Weekly.* https://www.usmagazine.com/celebrity-news/news/

giuliana-rancic-celebrates-being-five-years-cancer-free-w456639/ (accessed February 8, 2018).

Cleveland Clinic. "Chemotherapy Safety in the Home." Chemocare. com. http://chemocare.com/chemotherapy/side-effects/chemotherapy-safety.aspx (accessed May 15, 2018).

Cleveland Clinic. "Four Best Ways to Take Control of Abdominal Adhesions." Clevelandclinic.org. https://health.clevelandclinic. org/4-best-ways-to-take-control-of-abdominal-adhesions (accessed June 6, 2018).

Cleveland Clinic. "Four Heart Tests You May Need Before Cancer Treatment." Clevelandclinic.org. https://health.clevelandclinic. org/2014/11/4-heart-tests-you-may-need-before-cancer-treatment/ (accessed July 1, 2017).

Cleveland Clinic. "Treatment & Relief for Menopause & Hot Flashes." Clevelandclinic.org. https://my.clevelandclinic.org/health/ articles/15223-menopause-non-hormonal-treatment--relief-for-hot-flashes (accessed November 17, 2018).

Cochrane, Amanda. "Sharon Osbourne: Double Mastectomy Wasn't a Tough Decision." *CBS News*. https://www.cbsnews.com/news/sharon-osbourne-double-mastectomy-wasnt-a-tough-decision/ (accessed February 26, 2019).

Cohen, Robert. "Frequently Asked Post-Operative Questions." Scottsdale Center for Plastic Surgery. http://www.robertcohenmd. com/patient-resources/faq (accessed May 25, 2016).

Currin, Morag. "Microblading." Oncology Training International. http://oti-oncologytraining.com/2017/02/28/microblading/ (accessed July 14, 2018).

Davidson, Sara. "Crow's Nest: Interview with Sheryl Crow." *Reader's Digest*. http://www.rd.com/advice/relationships/crows-nest-interview-with-sheryl-crow/3/ (accessed December 14, 2016).

Dupere, Katie. "Betsey Johnson Kept Her Breast Cancer a Secret and She'd Do It Again." *Bustle.* www.bustle.com/p/betsey-johnson-kept-her-breast-cancer-a-secret-shed-do-it-again-79963 (accessed December 17, 2018).

Fernandez, Alexia. "Shannen Doherty Shows Off Growing Locks Two Months After She Announced Her Remission." *People.* http://people.com/style/shannen-doherty-growing-hair-after-remission-announcement/ (accessed September 19, 2017).

Fleishman, Stewart B., ed. "Understanding and Managing Chemotherapy Side Effects." CancerCare.org. https://www.cancer-care.org/publications/24 understanding and managing chemo-therapy side effects (accessed August 24, 2016).

Gardner, Stephanie S., ed. "Cosmetic Procedures: Scars." WebMD.com. https://www.webmd.com/beauty/cosmetic-procedures-scars (accessed June 6, 2018).

Gerstman, Leslie, "Microblading Eyebrow Restoration." Dr. Leslie Gerstman Laser and Cosmetic Medicine. https://drgerstman.com/eyebrow-microblading (accessed June 27, 2017).

Gerstner Sloan Kettering Graduate School of Biomedical Science. "Treatment for Lymphedema of the Legs." https://www.mskcc.org/cancer-care/patient-education/treatments-lymphedema-legs (accessed May 10, 2016).

Gibson, Amy. *Created Hair Designs.* Createdhair.com. https://www.createdhair.com/ (accessed December 14, 2018).

Gutsche, Kyla. "Tattooing that Transforms Appearances and Changes Lives." Cosmetic Transformations. http://www.cosmetictransforma-tions.com/ (accessed June 6, 2016).

Hider, Sarah. "The Power of Me: Choose Fearless." The Women's Fund of Central Ohio. http://www.womensfundcentralohio.

org/2015/02/12/power-of-me-choose-fearless/ (accessed December 14, 2016).

Hill, Jordan. "Diahann Carroll: 'It's My Responsibility to Help.'" BlackDoctor.org. https://blackdoctor.org/461431/diahann-caroll-its-my-responsibility-to-help-them/ (accessed February 26, 2019).

Institute for Quality and Efficiency in Health Care. "Oral Thrush: Prevention during Cancer Treatment." National Center for Biotechnology Information. www.ncbi.nlm.nih.gov/books/NBK367590/ (accessed May 18, 2016).

Javadian, Ani Nina. "Microblading: Dangers and Disasters." Ivy Laser Salon. http://www.ivylasersalon.com/microblading-dangers-and-disasters (accessed July 1, 2017).

Jordan, Julie. "Wanda Sykes: I Feel Whole Again." *People.* http://people.com/celebrity/wanda-sykes-breast-cancer-opens-up-about-double-mastectomy-healing/ (accessed December 14, 2016).

Laino, Charlene. "'Chemo Brain's Real, Not Just Patient's Imagination." *WebMD.* http://www.webmd.com/cancer/news/20121129/chemo-brain-real (accessed July 1, 2017).

Laughter Yoga International. "Laughter Yoga for Cancer." https://laughteryoga.org/laughter-yoga-for-cancer/ (accessed September 19, 2017).

Livestrong. "Ostomies." Livestrong.org. https://www.livestrong.org/we-can-help/finishing-treatment/ostomies (accessed October 3, 2016).

Mayo Clinic Staff. "Chemo Brain." Mayoclinic.org. http://www.mayoclinic.org/diseases-conditions/chemo-brain/home/ovc-20170224 (accessed July 1, 2017).

Mayo Clinic Staff. "Chemotherapy." Mayoclinic.org. https://www.mayoclinic.org/tests-procedures/chemotherapy/about/pac-20385033 (accessed August 29, 2016).

Mayo Clinic Staff. "Oral Thrush." Mayoclinic.org. https://www.mayoclinic.org/diseases-conditions/oral-thrush/symptoms-causes/syc-20353533 (accessed March 8, 2018).

Mayo Clinic Staff. "Ostomy: Adapting to Life after Colostomy, Ileostomy, or Urostomy." Mayoclinic.org. http://www.mayoclinic.org/diseases-conditions/colon-cancer/in-depth/ostomy/ART-20045825 (accessed January 27, 2017).

Meadows, Bob. "Christina Applegate Misses Her Old Breasts." *People.* http://people.com/tv/christina-applegate-misses-her-old-breasts/ (accessed December 14, 2016).

Minnesota Oncology. "Breast Cancer Treatment Options." https://mnoncology.com/disease-drug-info/types-of-cancer/breast-cancer/treatment-options/ (accessed Oct 11, 2018).

Moynihan, Timothy J. "Chemotherapy and Sex: Is Sexual Activity OK during Treatment?" Mayoclinic.org http://www.mayoclinic.org/tests-procedures/chemotherapy/expert-answers/chemotherapy-and-sex/faq-20058287 (accessed January 27, 2017).

Nash, Alanna. "Sheryl Crow and Melissa Etheridge Beat Breast Cancer and Heartbreak." *AARP The Magazine.* http://www.aarp.org/health/healthy-living/info-2014/sheryl-crow-melissa- etheridge-beat-cancer.html (accessed October 12, 2019).

National Cancer Institute. *Facing Forward: Life after Cancer Treatment.* https://www.cancer.gov/publications/patient-education/facing-forward (accessed September 19, 2017).

National Cancer Institute. "NCI Drug Dictionary." Cancer.gov. https://www.cancer.gov/publications/dictionaries/cancer-drug/def/soy-isoflavones (accessed November 17, 2018).

National Cancer Institute. "Prescribing Exercise as Cancer Treatment: A Conversation with Dr. Kathryn Schmitz." Cancer.gov. https://www.cancer.gov/news-events/cancer-currents-blog/2019/

cancer-survivors-exercise-guidelines-schmitz (accessed December 3, 2019).

National Comprehensive Cancer Network. "Exercise During Cancer Treatment." NCCN.org. https://www.nccn.org/patients/resources/life_with_cancer/exercise.aspx (accessed September 25, 2016).

"Nine Must-Haves Before You Start Chemo." *Beauty Over Cancer* (blog). https://beautyovercancer.wordpress.com/2009/10/18/eight-must-haves-before-you-start-chemo/ (accessed November 9, 2011).

Offenback, Mark S. "Dental Care for Cancer Patients: Before, During, and After Chemo or Radiation." WekivaDental.com. http://www.wekivadental.com/dental-care-cancer-patients-chemo-radiation/ (accessed May 6, 2019).

OncoLink Team. "Women's Guide to Sexuality During & After Cancer Treatment." OncoLink.org. https://www.oncolink.org/support/sexuality-fertility/sexuality/women-s-guide-to-sexuality-during-after-cancer-treatment (accessed May 11, 2019).

Organic Consumers Association. "How Toxic Are Your Household Cleaning Supplies?" *Green Guide.* https://www.organicconsumers.org/news/how-toxic-are-your-household-cleaning-supplies (accessed September 27, 2017).

Pelvic Exercises. "Hysterectomy Recovery Exercises for Recovering Strength and Fitness." PelvicExercises.com.au. https://www.pelvicexercises.com.au/safe-exercises-after-a-hysterectomy/ (accessed October 21, 2018).

Penguin Cold Caps. "Why Are So Many Chemotherapy Patients Choosing To Use the Penguin Cold Cap Therapy System?" Penguincoldcaps.com. https://penguincoldcaps.com/ (accessed June 22, 2016).

Prevent Cancer Infections. "Basic Hygiene Practices During Chemotherapy" PreventCancerInfections.org. September 20, 2018.

https://www.preventcancerinfections.org/health-tip-sheet/basic-hygiene-practices-during-chemotherapy# (accessed May 11, 2019).

Rawson, Rachel. "Caring for Scars after Breast Cancer Surgery." BreastCancerCare.org.uk. https://www.breastcancercare.org.uk/about-us/news-personal-stories/caring-scars-after-breast-cancer-surgery (accessed April 3, 2018).

Real, Evan. "Julia Louis-Dreyfus on Life after Breast Cancer Diagnosis: 'I'm Grateful.'" *The Hollywood Reporter*. https://www.hollywoodreporter.com/news/julia-louis-dreyfus-life-breast-cancer-diagnosis-1139702 (accessed September 4, 2018).

Roberts, Robin. "Wise Words from Robin Robert's Mom: 'Honey, Everybody's Got Something.'" NPR.org. https://www.npr.org/2014/04/27/306542402/wise-words-from-robin-roberts-mom-honey-everybody-s-got-something (accessed December 14, 2016).

Rockson, Stanley G., et al. "FAQs about Lymphedema." Lymphatic Education & Research Network. http://lymphaticnetwork.org/living-with-lymphedema/lymphedema/ (accessed August 24, 2016).

Salamon, Maureen. "Scarring and Breast Cancer Treatments." VeryWellHealth.com. https://www.verywellhealth.com/scarring-and-breast-cancer-430459 (accessed April 6, 2019).

Sea-Band. "Sea-Band FAQs." Sea-band.com. https://www.sea-band.com/faqs/ (accessed November 14, 2018).

Sholl, Jessie. "Eight Hidden Toxins: What's Lurking in Your Cleaning Products?" ExperienceLife.com. http://experiencelife.com/article/8-hidden-toxins-whats-lurking-in-your-cleaning-products/ (accessed September 21, 2017).

Shomon, Mary. "Ten Ways to Rock Your Thyroid Scar." HealthCentral.com. http://www.healthcentral.com/slideshow/how-to-rock-your-thyroid-scar (accessed January 9, 2018).

SLS Free. "Best Paraben Free Shampoo: Reviews of Three Amazing Brands." SLS Free. April 24, 2019. https://slsfree.net/paraben-free-shampoo-another-chemical-avoid/ (accessed May 14, 2019).

Susan G. Komen. "Lymphedema." Susan G. Komen. https://ww5.komen.org/BreastCancer/Lymphedema.html (accessed August 24, 2016).

Susan G. Komen. "Mastectomy." Susan G. Komen. http://ww5.komen.org/BreastCancer/MastectomyTheSurgicalProcedure.html (accessed August 26, 2016).

Theobald, Mikel. "How to Prepare for Chemotherapy." EverydayHealth.com. http://www.everydayhealth.com/cancer/how-to-prepare-for-chemotherapy-7064.aspx (accessed July 1, 2017).

Thompson Jr., Dennis. "When Cancer Changes Your Appearance." EverydayHealth.com. https://www.everydayhealth.com/cancer/when-cancer-changes-your-appearance.aspx (accessed September 19, 2017).

Thrash, Lee. "Sensible Solutions for Surgical Scars." Thebreastcaresite.com. http://www.thebreastcaresite.com/after-surgery/sensible-solutions-surgical-scars/ (accessed June 2, 2015).

Tronstad, Anne Katherine Aares. "Cold Gloves and Socks." *Oncolex Oncology Encyclopedia*. http://oncolex.org/Prosedyrer/TREATMENT/ComplicationTreatment/ColdGlovesSocks (accessed February 12, 2017).

UCSF Medical Center. "Diet for Cancer Treatment Side Effects." UCSFhealth.org. https://www.ucsfhealth.org/education/diet_for_cancer_treatment_side_effects (accessed October 27, 2018).

Us Weekly Staff. "Maura Tierney: 'I Was So Lucky' My Breast Cancer Was Detected Early." *Us Weekly*. https://www.usmagazine.com/celebrity-body/news/maura-tierney-parade-201099/ (accessed February 26, 2019).

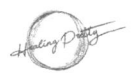

Vegan Ostomy. "VeganOstomy—Living with IBD and an Ostomy | Helping to Create Happy Ostomates" VeganOstomy.ca. https://www.veganostomy.ca/ (accessed May 11, 2019).

Weber, Douglas B. "Chemotherapy Treatments and Your Mouth." DWeberDDS. com https://www.dweberdds.com/chemotherapy-treatments-mouth/ (accessed August 22, 2018).

Whitlock, Jennifer. "How to Prevent or Minimize Surgery Scars." VeryWellHealth.com. https://www.verywellhealth.com/preventing-or-minimizing-scars-after-surgery-3156926 (accessed November 17, 2018).

Women Total Health & Wellness. "Look Good Feel Better® Care for Sensitive Skin during Treatment." MavenDoctors.io. https://mavendoctors.io/women/skin-beauty/look-good-feel-better-care-for-sensitive-skin-during-treatment-PgzWRuWPckK0B8T-VJ6gAw/ (accessed June 19, 2018).

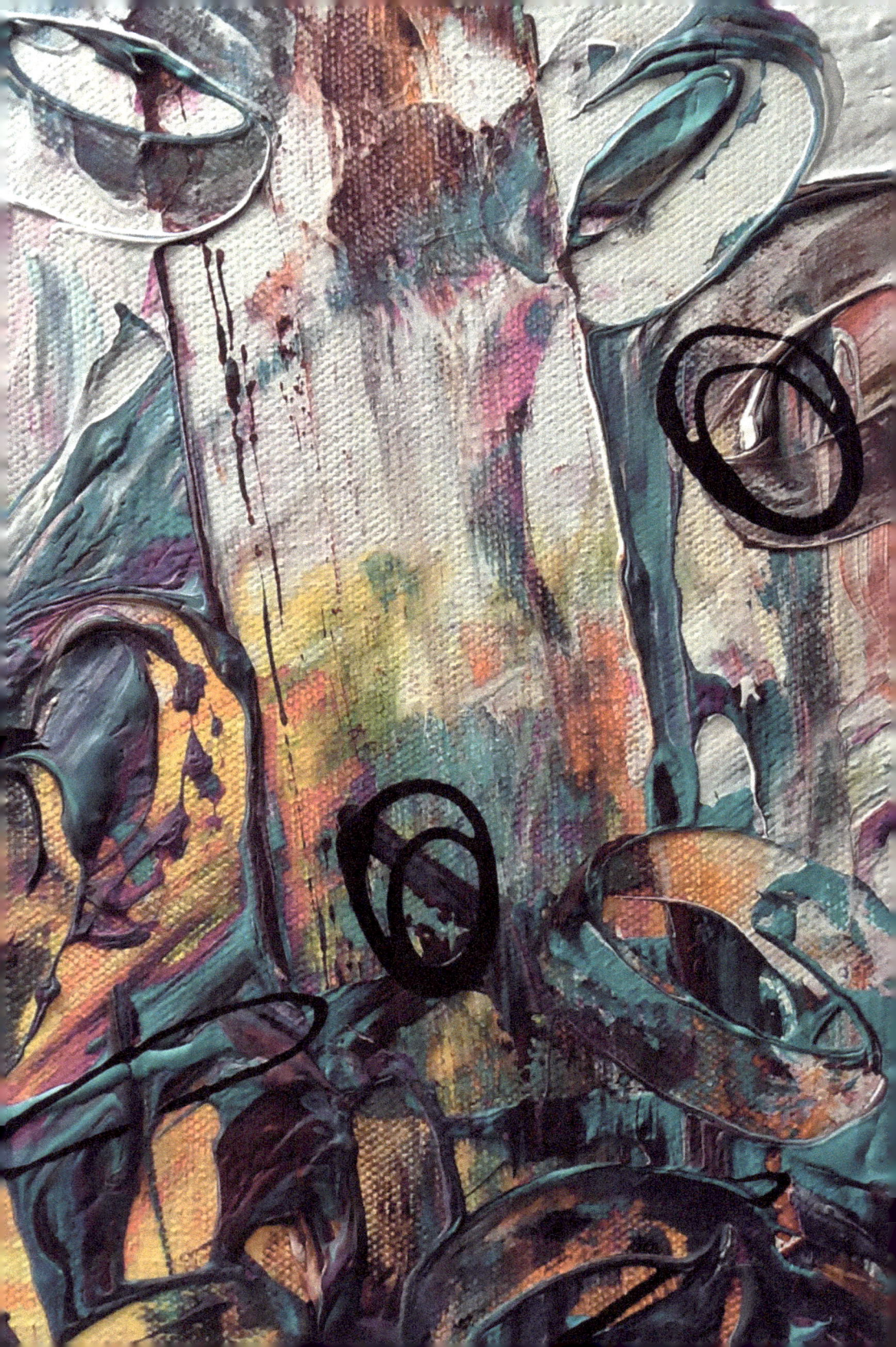

Notes & Journal

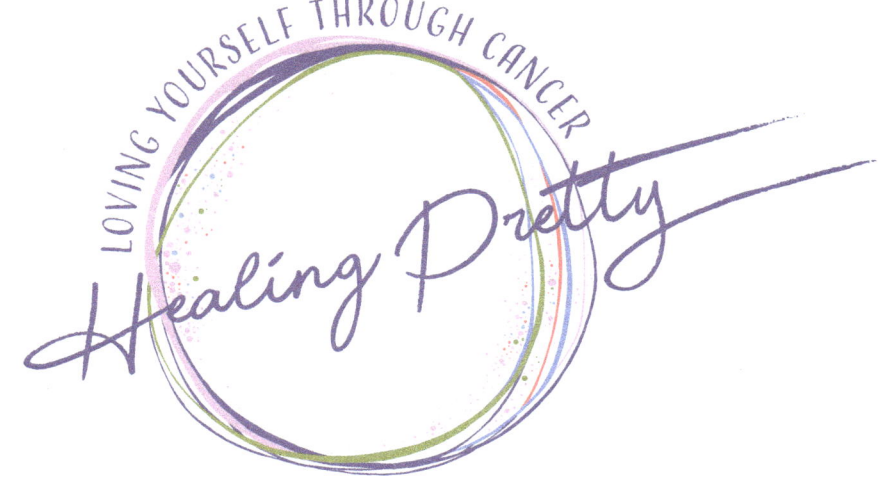

Could an organization or someone you know benefit from reading *Healing Pretty*? I am pleased to offer discounts on orders of 10 or more copies. You can reach me here:

Jackie@healingprettybook.com

www.healingprettybook.com

· · · · · · · · · · · · · ·

About the Author

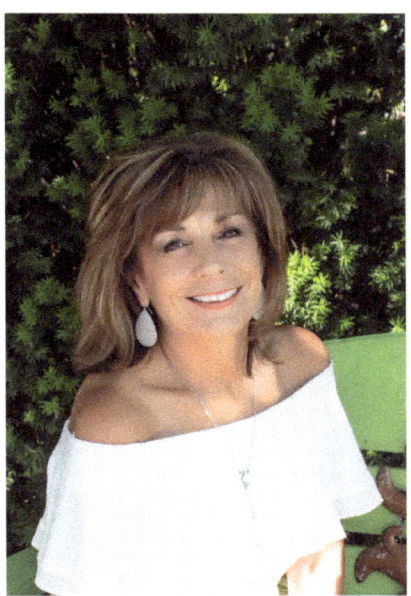

After supporting her beloved sister through lung and brain cancer, Jackie Apostol-Pizzuti realized her life's mission. She is trained and certified in skin, cosmetology, wig and mastectomy fitting for cancer patients, and has been a tirelessly dedicated volunteer at the International Look Good Feel Better® organization and her local cancer center for over ten years. She is the owner of Wigs to Wellness & The Mastectomy Boutique in Windsor, Ontario and continues to help thousands of women around the world discover choice, comfort, confidence, dignity, self-love, and healing on their roads to recovery.

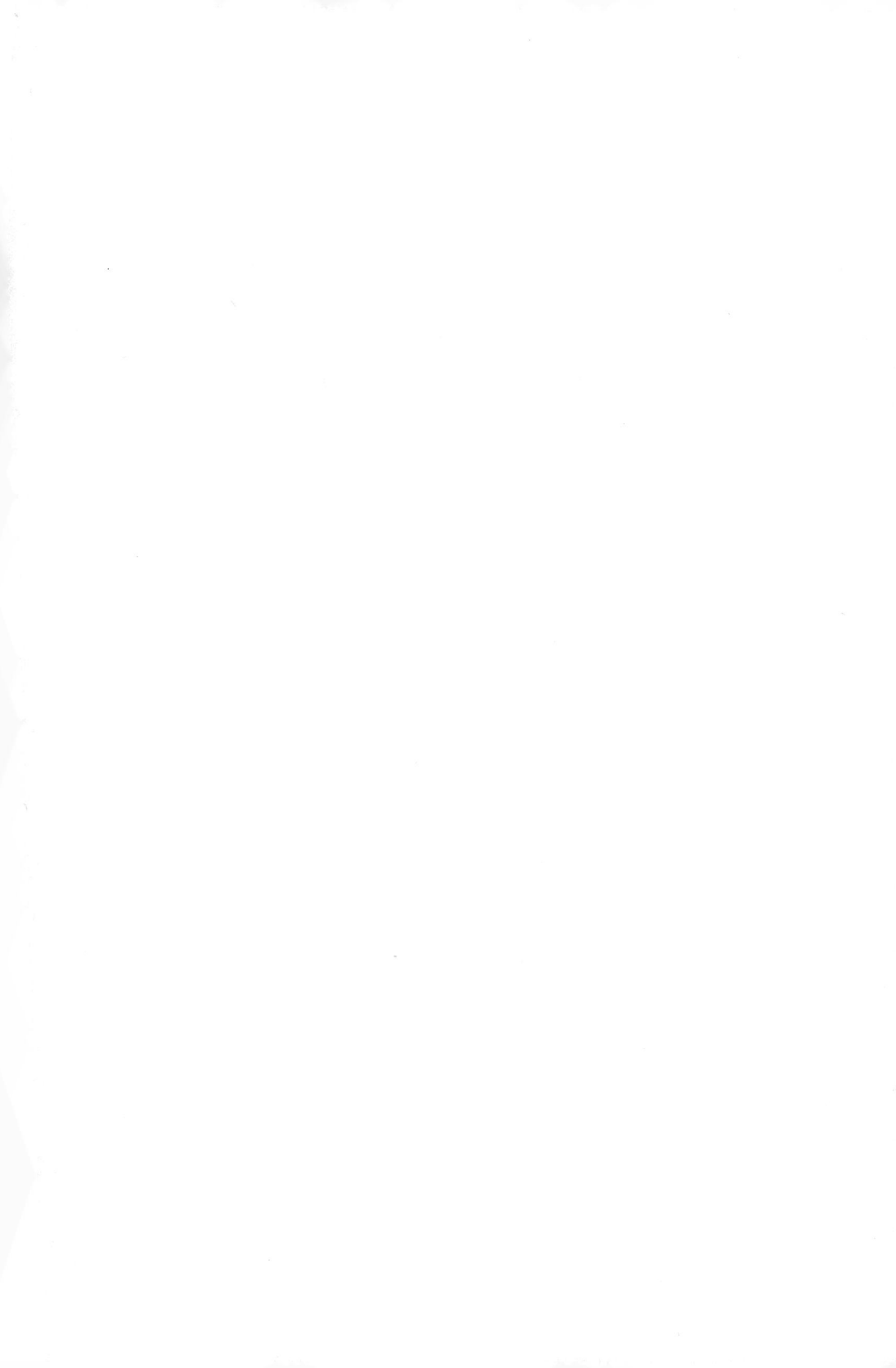

CPSIA information can be obtained
at www.ICGtesting.com
Printed in the USA
BVHW050533060820
585640BV00001B/1/J